LIVING WITH ALZHEIMER'S DISEASE

DR TOM SMITH has been writing full time since 1977, after spending six years in general practice and seven years in medical research. He writes the 'Doctor, Doctor' column in the *Guardian* on Saturdays, and also has ⟨illegible⟩ in the ⟨illegible⟩ *Carrick* ⟨illegible⟩. He has written two humorous books, *Doctor, Have You Got a Minute?* and *A Seaside Practice*, both published by Short Books. His other books for Sheldon Press include *Heart Attacks: Prevent and Survive, Coping Successfully with Prostate Cancer, Overcoming Back Pain, Coping with Bowel Cancer, Coping with Heartburn and Reflux, Coping with Age-Related Memory Loss, Skin Cancer: Prevent and Survive, How to Get the Best from Your Doctor* and *Coping with Kidney Disease*.

Overcoming Common Problems Series

Selected titles
A full list of titles is available from Sheldon Press,
36 Causton Street, London SW1P 4ST, and on our website at
www.sheldonpress.co.uk

Overcoming Common Problems Series

Overcoming Common Problems Series

Overcoming Common Problems

Living with Alzheimer's Disease

Dr Tom Smith

sheldon **PRESS**

First published in Great Britain in 2000

Sheldon Press
36 Causton Street
London SW1P 4ST

Second new edition published 2004

Copyright © Dr Tom Smith 2000, 2004

The author and publisher have made every effort to ensure that the
external website and email addresses included in this book are correct
and up to date at the time of going to press. The author and
publisher are not responsible for the content, quality or
continuing accessibility of the sites.

British Library Cataloguing-in-Publication Data
A catalogue record for this book is available from the British Library

ISBN 978–0–85969–956–3

3 5 7 9 10 8 6 4 2

Typeset by Deltatype Limited, Birkenhead, Merseyside
Printed in Great Britain by Ashford Colour Press

Produced on paper from sustainable forests

For Angus and Craig

Contents

Abbreviations

ACEI	angiotensin-converting enzyme inhibitor
ACTH	adrenocorticotrophic hormone
ADAS-cog	Alzheimer's Disease Assessment Scale cognitive subscale
ADAS-noncog	Alzheimer's Disease Assessment Scale non-cognitive subscale
ADCS	Alzheimer's Disease Cooperative Study
ADCS-CGIC	Alzheimer's Disease Cooperative Study – Clinical Global Impression Change
ADL	activities of daily living
AIDS	acquired immune deficiency syndrome
ApoC	apo lipoprotein C
ApoE	apo lipoprotein E
APP	amyloid precursor protein
BEHAVE-AD	Behavioural Pathology in Alzheimer's Disease
BPRS	Brief Psychiatric Rating Scale
BRSD	Behaviour Rating Scale for Dementia
CarenapD	Care Needs Assessment Pack for Dementia
CARET	Beta-Carotene and Retinol Efficacy Trial
CDR	Clinical Dementia Rating
CERAD	Consortium to Establish a Registry for Alzheimer's Disease
CGI	Clinical Global Impression
CIBIC	Clinicians' Interview-Based Impression of Change
CJD	Creuzfeldt-Jakob disease
CMAI	Cohen-Mansfield Agitation Inventory
CSF	cerebrospinal fluid
CT	computer-assisted tomography
DADS	Disability Assessment in Dementia Scale
DOPA	dihydroxyphenylalanine
ECT	electroconvulsant treatment
EEG	electro-encephalography
FDA	Food and Drugs Administration
GABA	gamma aminobutyric acid
GDS	Global Deterioration Scale
GMS	Geriatric Mental State Examination

HRT	hormone replacement therapy
IADL	Instrumental Activities of Daily Living
ICM	Information-Concentration-Memory test
IU	International Unit
MMSE	Mini Mental State Examination
MRI	magnetic resonance imaging
NGF	nerve growth factor
NPI	Neuropsychiatric Inventory
NYU	New York University
PDS	Progressive Deterioration Scale
PET	positron emission tomography
PSMS	Physical Self-Maintenance Scale
SCAG	Sandoz Clinical Assessment Geriatric
SIB	Severe Impairment Battery
SKT	Syndrom Kurztest
SPECT	single proton emission computed tomography
WHO	World Health Organization

Introduction

I have on my desk as I write this a letter from a 59-year-old schoolteacher. She writes:

> I have just been given the news that I have early Alzheimer's disease. I went to my doctor because I haven't been getting on well in school – forgetting things, being a bit muddled sometimes, that sort of thing – and I thought it was just my age. But tests show that it's Alzheimer's. As you can imagine, I'm shocked beyond belief. What lies ahead of me? Will I be able to cope for at least a while? Is there anything I can do myself to improve my outlook? Or do I face a hopeless decline into senseless oblivion? Please be honest with me.

I had been thinking about writing this book for a while, but her letter has forced my hand. What follows is dedicated to that brave woman, and to the many patients with this devastating disease I have helped to care for over the years. It is also dedicated to the people who have looked after them – relatives, friends, nurses and professional carers. And there is a third group to whom I pay huge tribute – the people who have given us hope in our struggle against the dementias: the research scientists who have finally developed medicines that can slow down the relentless progression of the disease. I report many medical meetings: my conversations with the experts at meetings on Alzheimer's disease have convinced me that it will eventually be defeated.

Sadly, such a cure is out of the reach, for the moment, of my schoolteacher friend. Because she is in the early stages, still with insight into her problems, and able to run her own life reasonably efficiently, we can give her drugs to slow down her deterioration. We can organize many aspects of her life to help her remain as independent as she can be. And we can plan ahead with her and her family for the more difficult times. This book is about how all this can be done for anyone with dementia.

The need for better treatments for dementia is extremely urgent.

Today there are 750,000 people in Britain with dementia, and more than 400,000 of them are classified as having Alzheimer's disease. The numbers are set to rise further as we become a more aged society. For the first time in history, the over-60s outnumber the under-16s in Britain, and the number of those with dementia is expected to rise to about 840,000 by 2010 and to more than 1.5 million by 2050.

These figures are not peculiar to Britain – they apply to every developed country. Dementia is ubiquitous, and will be the main public health problem in the new millennium. People with dementia already occupy half of all hospital and nursing home beds in North America: four million Europeans already need daily care because of dementia, and the figure is rising annually. This clearly puts an immense burden on health resources and costs. Dementia in old age is the main reason for the British National Health Service no longer being free to the elderly people who are chronically ill and need nursing care. They must sell their homes and their finances must be run down to very low levels before the state will help them. In the United States, many elderly people die in poverty, their homes sold and their relatives running out of money to support them. In Germany the costs of health care for the elderly are now compulsorily visited upon grandchildren and even great-grand-children. And as the ratio of the workforce to the retired population becomes smaller, year by year, this huge burden will increase.

Thus, we have to be prepared to look after our elderly ill relatives ourselves, in the home. There will only be nursing home and hospital care for the very few, and for those whose disease is so advanced that it can no longer be managed outside a residential environment. The families of people with dementia must face the fact that there may be many years ahead when they must care for their sick relatives themselves.

This book is about how to make those years as comfortable and bearable as possible for people with dementia and their carers. It maps out the usual course of dementia, from diagnosis to end-care. Not all people follow the same path at the same speed, but the pattern of developing dementia is broadly similar. This book spells out the milestones, the problems to be expected, and how they can best be faced.

If this sounds profoundly depressing, the book is not entirely pessimistic. There is a new optimism among researchers. Knowledge of the origins of dementia has grown, and new ideas on how to control it and even perhaps to reverse its progression have brought medicines specifically for dementia closer to the medical market. These advances, and what the future may bring, are gradually emerging from the laboratory towards the clinic. Those that are showing promise now – in mid-2004 – are explained in this edition. I confidently expect that by 2008 some of them will already be in daily use, and that there will be other approaches developed that we cannot yet predict. Things are moving very fast in dementia research, and this book can only scratch the surface of what is going on behind the scenes.

A quite separate source of my optimism about the future care of people with dementia is the growth of voluntary societies and organizations prepared to help sufferers and their carers. At last carers are getting the appreciation they deserve. Health authorities, too, are beginning to recognize how important it is to support them. This book will describe in detail all the ways in which carers can get help, and how they can get in touch with those who provide that help.

This book is mainly about Alzheimer's disease, because this is the cause of most dementias in the elderly. It is a primary disorder of the brain nerve cells. But there are other causes of dementia; among them are the following:

- multi-infarct disease, caused by a series of small strokes;
- Pick's disease, which is inherited and affects the front part of the brain so that people with it lose their judgement and inhibitions;
- Huntington's disease, also inherited, which first affects people's movements before leading to a rapid dementia in middle age;
- Creuzfeldt-Jakob disease, or CJD, which of course is very well known as the human form of 'mad cow disease';
- dementias related to AIDS, alcohol abuse, drug abuse and traumas.

They are all given their place in these pages, particularly because the care of people with these diseases is similar to that of Alzheimer's sufferers. This list is obviously very depressing, as most of us are well aware of how poor the outlook is for most of these diseases. So I should add an optimistic note here. Alzheimer's disease is not the end of the world. There are many ways in which its effects can be ameliorated, and most people with it can be helped to enjoy a reasonable quality of life. It is not an immediate sentence of death, and many families in which there is a case of Alzheimer's can, with help, enjoy much of what lies ahead of them.

1
Defining dementia

In these days of computerization and collection of data for research purposes and payment of medical bills, whether by the state or by medical insurance systems, every disease must have its definition, and dementia is no exception. Every few years the World Health Organization and the American Psychiatric Association review and update their definitions of dementia. This process should, over the years, have made the diagnosis of dementia clearer. I leave it to readers to decide whether they have been successful.

The latest definition of dementia formulated by the American psychiatrists runs as follows:

(A) Multiple cognitive deficits manifested by both:
   (1) memory impairment and
   (2) at least one of the following cognitive disturbances:
      (a) aphasia
      (b) apraxia
      (c) agnosia
      (c) disturbance in executive functioning
(B) The cognitive deficits cause significant impairment in social or occupational function and represent decline from a previous functional level

The World Health Organization (WHO) uses plainer language. Its definition of dementia runs as follows:

Presence of each of the following:

- A decline in memory which causes impaired functioning in daily living.
- A decline in intellectual abilities:
  Deterioration in thinking and in the processing of information, of a degree leading to impaired functioning in daily living.
- No clouding of consciousness, such as sleepiness, drowsiness, etc.
- A deterioration in emotional control, social behaviour or motivation.

1

- Symptoms should have clearly been present for at least six months.

Both definitions stress that there is loss of both intellect (understanding, or cognition) and of memory, and that there are also changes in emotions and behaviour. By cognitive deficits the American psychiatrists mean loss of aspects of knowledge and understanding that the patient would normally have, such as the ability to follow and take a constructive part in a conversation. That daily crossword is often the first to go when dementia begins.

Yet some skills may be retained long after others are lost. I play golf regularly with John, a man in his seventies who is so far along the road of his Alzheimer's dementia that he has lost most of his conversation. Yet, given the right club in his hand, he can still play to a handicap of 18. He cannot follow his ball in flight, nor can he add up his score, and he has to have his putts lined up for him – but he can still sink them better than I can.

John is fortunate that he has many old friends who take it in turn to transport him between golf course and home, and give his wife a well-earned rest. Although he no longer knows their names, or, for that matter, his own, he still clearly takes pleasure in their company. He conforms to the American psychiatrists' definition of dementia in that he obviously has aphasia (can no longer speak, despite still possessing the normal mechanisms in the throat to do so). He also has agnosia (he does not recognize or easily identify everyday objects – except his golf clubs and balls). Strictly, he does not have apraxia (inability to carry out physical actions, despite having normal muscle structure and function) because he has retained his golf swing. But he certainly has disturbed executive function – he can no longer plan or organize the simplest actions, even including the next shot at his beloved game. That has to be planned for him. All he has to do is to use his swing.

What is clearest of all about John is that he conforms closely to part (B) of the American psychiatrists' definition, and all the sections of the WHO definition, of dementia. He is a long way down the road of dementia, having had it for at least ten years, yet he is still reasonably happy, and with the help of his friends, he and his wife can have a bearable life.

We know that John has Alzheimer's-type dementia, because hospital investigations several years ago gave us the diagnosis, and his gradual deterioration since then has confirmed it. But what about my schoolteacher friend? Do we assume that she has Alzheimer's after a short visit to her doctor? Even if the symptoms fit with the WHO definition above? Not necessarily.

Professor Timo Erkinjuntti, of the Memory Research Unit at the University of Helsinki, and President of the Finnish Alzheimer Association, sees as a major challenge the need to defend every person's rights to an accurate diagnosis of memory and dementia disorders. He believes that too often the patient's and the carer's complaints are ignored by medical professionals, and that the modern customer, the patient, should not accept old-fashioned attitudes. One of these attitudes is to accept as an Alzheimer's case a patient who fulfils the WHO criteria without further tests and investigations.

Timo objects to this because such a diagnosis is so final, when the memory loss and loss of intellect may be due to another, and even reversible, cause. For example, temporary problems with memory may be caused by multiple minor strokes (such as transient ischaemic attacks, described later), epilepsy, abuse of drugs and alcohol, minor brain injuries, and some psychiatric illnesses, particularly depression. Thyroid underactivity ('myxoedema') is also a major cause of dementia-like symptoms in older people.

Less common, but just as reversible, causes of dementia include vitamin B12 deficiency (in which the dementia occurs along with pernicious anaemia), and conditions within the brain such as abscesses, benign tumours, old bruising after a minor head injury ('subdural haematoma'), and excess fluid pressure within the brain ('hydrocephalus'). Some medicines (mainly sedatives, tranquillizers and/or anti-convulsants) may produce dementia-like symptoms, as can chronic poisons, such as prolonged and excessive contact with certain industrial and agricultural chemicals, such as lead and organo-phosphates. Sadly, we may see many more cases of dementia if predictions about the long-term after-effects of Ecstasy are correct. They will not be reversible.

So, to make the diagnosis of Alzheimer's disease, it is incumbent on doctors to rule out all these possibly reversible causes of dementia first, and if they are found, to start the reversal. That is easy, and dramatic, in the case of myxoedema or of B12 deficiency, in which the diagnosis may even be made by a careful physical examination and confirmed by a simple blood test. But the routine investigation of a new case of suspected dementia in many cases does need very specialized neurological tests, such as brain scans, before the final diagnosis of Alzheimer's can be made with certainty. These investigations are described in Chapter 4.

So what would I recommend to my schoolteacher friend? I would first find out if she had had all the investigations to rule out other causes of her dementia before fully accepting the diagnosis. I know she was in a car crash a few months ago. Could that have left her with an unexpected head injury? Did she have her thyroid and B12 levels measured? Has she had other symptoms that don't quite fit with early Alzheimer's disease, like headaches, blurred vision, or signs of nerve problems in a particular site, like a limb, that might suggest a possibly reversible brain problem? She is relatively young for Alzheimer's – has a close relative also suffered with early onset dementia? If not, could the diagnosis be wrong? If I were her, I would pull out all the stops to make sure the diagnosis is correct before accepting it. That may involve going as far as to arrange brain scans to confirm or rule out the disease.

In the meantime, she wants to know what causes Alzheimer's – she is still curious about the processes going on inside her. What I would tell her is in Chapter 2.

2

Understanding Alzheimer's

In 1906 Dr Alois Alzheimer, who lived in Germany from 1864 to 1915, reported on the microscopic findings in the brain of a woman who had died from what he considered a rare mental illness. Her first symptom had been an unreasonable and overwhelming jealousy. It was soon followed by memory problems, and two months later by apraxia (see pages 1, 2). She became nervous and could not organize her household money. She assumed that the conversations of everyone around her were about her. She deteriorated quickly into complete dementia.

Some idea of Dr Alzheimer's meticulous attention to detail is given by Figure 2.1, taken from the post-mortem microscopic examination of this unfortunate woman's brain. Alzheimer described two main deviations from the normal brain. The first was that many of the 'neurofibrils', structures that normally extend out from nerve cells like the spreading branches of a tree, and which we now know pass on the nerve messages from each cell to the others around it, are tangled. They criss-cross each other in a haphazard way, and their endings are not in close contact with the neurofibrils of the other, adjacent, cells. Such tangles obviously mean that the affected cells are no longer communicating with the rest of the brain.

The second was the presence of areas, or 'plaques', of 'amyloid', a strange smooth-looking material without visible internal structure between and around the brain cells, that often appears to replace the cells, taking up much of the space that the cells would otherwise occupy.

For many years it was accepted that the combination of neurofibrillary tangles and amyloid plaques was the definitive sign, at post-mortem, that the patient had had Alzheimer's disease. It was not known whether amyloid plaques actually caused damage to brain cells or were a scar-type reaction to dying brain cells, but it seemed obvious that they were closely linked with damaged brain cells. The tangles were assumed to be a sign that the surviving brain cells were disorganized and could not perform their function of passing on messages from one part of the brain to another. They were known to be associated with the amyloid plaques – they were almost always

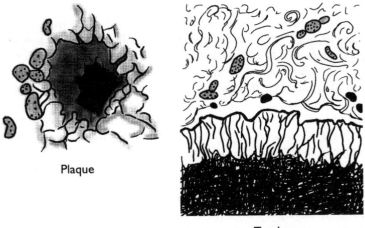

Plaque

Tangles

Figure 2.1 The histopathology of Alzheimer's disease – From Alzheimer's own case in *The Early Story of Alzheimer's Disease*. Edited by K. L. Bick, L. Amaducci and G. Pepeu (1987)

found together. Could the presence of the amyloid be causing the tangles, or vice versa, or were the two mutually dependent on some as yet unknown inflammatory process common to them both? If we could find out why these two changes were occurring, we might find ways to stop them and even possibly reverse the process.

However, as research continued it became clear that Alzheimer's is not the only disease with tangles and plaques: they occur in other brain disorders (such as Down's syndrome and Creuzfeldt-Jakob disease), and they are sometimes found incidentally at post-mortem in people who have not had dementia. They are certainly a sign of an abnormal process in the brain, but whether they are a cause, or a result, of the symptoms remains the subject of academic debate.

I say academic, because such changes are found only at post-mortem, so that knowledge of them is hardly of any practical use to living patients. But the research stimulated by the discovery of plaques and tangles has produced results that are now being translated into practical developments in diagnosis during life and in treatment that actually makes a difference. These results have come from people in medical disciplines as different as genetics, biochemistry, brain imaging, and microbiology, all working together.

The genetics of Alzheimer's

As mentioned in the Introduction, dementia commonly accompanies advancing age all over the world. However, that rule doesn't necessarily mean that all over the world Alzheimer's is the commonest form of dementia. Nor does Alzheimer's follow the same pattern in every country. For example, in a WHO review of dementia, A. S. Henderson reported that some researchers had found it to be more common in women than in men in some regions of their countries, such as Turku, in Finland, in Rochester, in the United States, and in Italy. In Britain, Sweden, Japan, and the rest of Finland, however, the disease attacked the sexes in equal numbers.

Different areas of the world seem to attract different forms of dementia. For example, Alzheimer's is much commoner than dementia due to multiple small strokes (vascular dementia) in most of Europe and North America, but in China, Japan, and Russia the reverse is the case. And even within Europe, the French, Germans and Italians have much higher numbers of cases of vascular dementia per head of population than Britain, the Netherlands and Scandinavia. They may reflect differences in local environments that make people more or less susceptible than elsewhere to the different types of dementia, or they may just be due to the ways doctors diagnose dementia, and not be a real difference.

The figures do not explain, however, why Alzheimer's is apparently extremely rare among the Cree Indians of North America, and may even not occur at all in Nigeria. (This last piece of information comes from the Henderson WHO report and is astonishing if true.) These variations among and between populations may be explained, at least in part, by genetic differences. Could people be protected against, or predisposed to, dementia by their inheritance – their genetic make-up? Are there families in which there are far more cases of Alzheimer's than would be expected to happen by chance? Naturally, this is a very important question: when a new case of Alzheimer's is diagnosed the first thought that comes into every close relative's mind, whether it is voiced or not, is 'will I get this disease?'

The answers are provided by the WHO report I have already mentioned. A history of dementia in a first-degree relative (parent, brother or sister) increases our chances of dementia by between two and five times. Don't be too upset by this – it means, as dementia is a relatively rare illness in people under 80 years old, that you still have a very small chance of developing it until you are very old. There are a very few families in which Alzheimer's is inherited as a dominant gene, so that their members' chances of developing it eventually are around one in two – but they can be counted on the fingers of one hand among the populations of most European countries.

An exception to these rules is the presence of Down's syndrome. Nearly all people with Down's syndrome develop, by the time they reach their thirties, the amyloid plaques and neurofibrillary tangles typical of the brain changes in Alzheimer's (see page 5). At the same time, they develop an Alzheimer's-type dementia. There is evidence that some people with a close relative with Down's syndrome are also at higher risk of Alzheimer's.

Why should this be? One clue is to be found on chromosome 21. Chromosomes are the strings of proteins on which we 'thread' our genes, of which we have many thousands. Genes produce the characteristics which make us what we are – eye and hair colour, height, much of our appearance, our immune system, and so on. We have 23 pairs of 'somatic' chromosomes (which determine non-sexual characteristics) and one pair of chromosomes (labelled XX in the case of women and XY in the case of men) that determine, among other things, our gender.

The mutation in the gene that leads to Down's syndrome is found in a specific position on chromosome 21: it lies immediately beside another that causes early onset Alzheimer's (starting around the age of 50 or younger). The link between Down's syndrome and Alzheimer's dementia is that the mutation may involve the whole segment of the chromosome that involves both genes: people with one mutation are more likely than normal to possess the other one, too.

The geneticists have linked at least three other genetic faults with Alzheimer's: two that, like the fault on chromosome 21, predispose their owner to early onset dementia are found on chromosomes 1 and 14. They are very rare. Much more common is a fault with chromosome 19, which gives rise to late onset Alzheimer's disease (i.e. that arises after the age of 60).

This fault in chromosome 19 was a vital clue to one underlying biochemical fault in Alzheimer's. That particular gene is instrumental in producing a substance (a compound of fat and protein) called apo lipoprotein E, or ApoE. There are several types of ApoE, according to their chemistry. Inheriting one of them, ApoE4, from both parents (giving a 'double ApoE4') was linked with a 17.9-fold increase in a person's risk of Alzheimer's disease. Several studies since have shown that many of the differences in dementia cases in populations could be put down to the proportion of them who possess a double ApoE4 in their genetic make-up.

In fact, there is now good evidence that possessing double ApoE4 makes us more susceptible than normal to a poor memory as we age, irrespective of whether we develop dementia. In Helsinki, Professor Paavo Riekkinen of the University of Kuopio reported that older people with ApoE4 have a poorer long-term memory than people with ApoE2 or ApoE3.

The scientists are beginning to unravel the secrets of chromosomes 14 and 21, too. They are studying 'heat shock proteins', the genes for which are located on chromosome 14, and amyloid precursor protein (APP) made by a gene on chromosome 21, as other possible contributors to dementia. And they have not given up on chromosome 19, where yet another gene, the one that makes apo lipoprotein C (ApoC) may also be involved in the disease.

None of these findings mean that people worried that they might develop Alzheimer's should rush to get genetic testing. There are 100-year-old people with double ApoE4 who are completely normal for their age – so that there must be other underlying causes that spark off the disease. And there are people with Alzheimer's disease who possess none of these 'rogue' genes. However, they are a pointer on which to base research, particularly in establishing in people with dementia the changes in their body's chemistry, arrest of which may lead eventually to treatment and reversal of their dementia.

The chemistry of Alzheimer's

The acetylcholine story

One target of the biochemical teams has been 'neurotransmitters'. These are the chemical 'messengers' that pass on messages between brain cells. Every brain cell manufactures and secretes into the space around it a chemical transmitter that stirs the cell next to it into action. They are the basis of memory, reason, emotion, mood, alertness or sleepiness, sexual arousal, aggression, physical activity, even consciousness itself. In fact, they underlie everything we sense and do.

In the last few years we have unravelled the mechanisms and structures of many brain neurotransmitters. We know how they are disturbed in depression, and from that knowledge we have developed extremely efficient antidepressant drugs that control the concentrations in the brain of the neurotransmitters noradrenaline and serotonin. The same goes for a disease closely linked to Alzheimer's disease, Parkinson's disease, in which the neurotransmitter DOPA (a chemical transmitter in the brain related to adrenaline) is disturbed. DOPA and GABA are neurotransmitters – chemicals that pass between brain cells. They and other neurotransmitters like them can alter mood, speed up thought, process memory and help to control muscles, voluntary (as in the limbs) or involuntary (as in the lungs, heart and gut).

The breakthrough in Alzheimer's was the discovery that even in the early stages, the brains of Alzheimer's patients were low in their level of the neurotransmitter acetylcholine. Acetylcholine seems to be the main neurotransmitter between the nerves that provide us with learning and memory and behaviour patterns – and these are the three main problems in Alzheimer's disease.

The evidence that acetylcholine is crucial to Alzheimer's comes from three sources. The first two are in animals and the third in people with the disease. First, drugs can be used in animal models to increase the amount of free acetylcholine in the brain. When the level is raised the animals are livelier and better able to deal with complicated mazes to get at food – a test of animal 'intelligence' and memory.

Second, when the cells in the brain of animals that produce acetylcholine are damaged, the animals become demented. Their learning defects and poor memory are both reversed after transplants into their brains of fetal nerve cells or other cells that restore their brain acetylcholine levels.

Third, as we age we gradually lose our acetylcholine-producing brain cells. This is a normal part of ageing: it is nothing to worry about, because most of us still have plenty of acetylcholine sloshing about in our brains even when we die in extreme old age. However, this process is greatly accelerated in Alzheimer's, regardless of the age at which it starts, and the severity of dementia is directly related to the falling brain acetylcholine levels. Dementia is not just accelerated ageing – it is a disease quite separate from normal ageing, and if the loss of acetylcholine can be arrested or even reversed at an early stage, there should be tremendous benefit for the patient. The problem still facing the researchers and doctors is how best to stop this loss. How we are trying to do so at the moment is described in Chapter 3.

However, to think of acetylcholine alone as the answer to Alzheimer's is, sadly, too simplistic. The Alzheimer's brain may have other faults, too. One may be the way it deals with the mineral, calcium.

The calcium story

Brain cells, to function normally, have to have exactly the right amount of calcium inside them. Calcium is at the centre of many processes inside the cell, including the use of its energy stores and the production and secretion of neurotransmitters. These vital processes are disturbed if the cell is overloaded with calcium.

The passage of calcium from the tissue fluid outside the cells into them is finely tuned by calcium 'channels' in their outer membrane. This mechanism goes crucially wrong when the brain is injured, as after an accident or a stroke. In these circumstances, the cell membrane does not function correctly, the channels open up, and calcium flows freely into the cell. This high level of calcium stops many vital processes inside the cell, which then dies.

There are drugs that block the calcium channels on the surface of brain cells – not unreasonably they are called calcium channel blockers – so that they prevent the build-up of calcium inside the cells. So far their benefit has been proved in people who have had a particular type of bleeding into the brain, called subarachnoid haemorrhage, so much so that one calcium channel blocker in particular, nimodipine, is now the standard emergency treatment for the condition. People given it immediately after a subarachnoid haemorrhage have much less residual brain damage, including dementia, than those who do not receive it. A very large trial of nimodipine, to be given as soon as possible after a stroke, is taking place, in which around a quarter of all Dutch general practitioners are taking part.

However, trials of calcium channel blockers have not proved successful in long-term dementia – perhaps because they are not specific enough for the brain. Most of them also act on the blood pressure and the heart and the rest of the circulation, and that may not be desirable in dementia. Nimodipine is only the start: we can expect even more brain-specific calcium channel blockers in the future.

The inflammation story

To acetylcholine and calcium must be added the chemistry of inflammation. First, I should explain what inflammation is. It is the body's reaction to an attack on the tissues. The attack might be an infection, from a virus or a bacterium, for instance. A boil on the skin and the common cold are examples. With a boil, the redness and swelling of the skin, the collection of pus and the boil's eventual healing, perhaps leaving a small scar, are all part of the process of inflammation. The infecting organism, in this case the bacterium *Staphylococcus aureus*, stimulates the body to send extra blood to the affected region (hence the swelling and redness); the blood contains white cells and antibodies that will kill the germs. The pus, a mixture of the white cells and the remains of the dead germs and tissues, is the result of the battle between the body's defences and the bacteria. The scar is the body's way of healing the disrupted skin.

A cold is a similar inflammatory reaction, but to one of the many viruses that can invade the sensitive layer of cells lining the nose and throat. The redness and swelling lead to congestion (the stuffy feeling) inside the nose, which is usually followed by the production of a lot of mucus (the pus) and the resolution – the return of the nose to normal.

However, a germ such as a bacterium or a virus is not always present in an inflammatory response. The inflammation may be a sign that the body has reacted in an abnormal way to such an invasion in the past, and that this abnormal reaction has caused the immune system to start to destroy normal tissues. Such a disease is termed an 'auto-immune' disease. It is well known to play a part in common diseases like rheumatoid arthritis, thyroid disease and in-flammatory bowel disease (like Crohn's disease or ulcerative colitis).

Evidence of the link between inflammation and Alzheimer's
In 2000, when I wrote the first edition of this book, there were only hints, and little evidence, that inflammation of the brain might be the starting point and the continuing reason for its steady deterioration in Alzheimer's disease. However, this theory was suspected to be true because biochemical tests on the brains of Alzheimer's sufferers had shown 'markers' of inflammation, as if an infective agent had stimulated the brain's immune response. The markers include:

- substances known as cytokines, which appear in many inflammatory diseases;
- the deposition of a complex chemical, 'complement', that is usually instrumental in removing invading germs by the white blood cells;
- the activation of 'microglial' cells in the brain. Microglia are the scar tissue of the brain, much like the scar tissue that appears after a wound in the skin.

Now, however, we have the evidence that there is a strong link between all the processes that cause inflammation and Alzheimer's. A leading article in the *British Medical Journal* (*BMJ*) (pages 1139–46) spells out the facts, particularly with regard to the link between cholesterol and inflammation, and drugs called statins (see below). Its complex medical language makes it hard going for non-medical readers, so I will present a summary of its main messages in layman's terms here and on pages 65–68. What the article has to say will be the basis of much more research in the near future, and will lead to medicines and approaches to the disease that are more effective than those currently available. In fact, the findings in the article are already showing practical benefits. Written by Ivan Cassidy and Eric Topol of the Cleveland Clinic in the USA, this review of 468 scientific reports is the most comprehensive explanation to date of the causes and future treatments of Alzheimer's disease.

Cholesterol, inflammation and statins
Types of inflammation, such as those seen in a boil and the common cold, are readily understood, but there is another form that arises not

from an infection, but from the body's reaction to chemicals naturally circulating within it. The substance that has received most attention in the last decade or so, and with which you will be most familiar, is cholesterol. Although cholesterol is a chemical normally found in the body (it is a means of distributing fat to the tissues), too much of it in the bloodstream can lead to disease.

Classically, too much cholesterol can result in fatty degeneration of the arteries or 'atheroma'. Atheroma is named after the Greek word for porridge; collections of cholesterol in the walls of arteries in the heart (the coronary arteries) and in the brain (the cerebral arteries) give the artery walls a porridge-like consistency. If not treated, these deposits of atheroma lead to strokes and heart attacks. In the 1990s it was shown beyond doubt that lowering the levels of cholesterol in blood significantly decreases the risk of a stroke or heart attack. Proof of this fact is the huge fall in strokes and heart attacks in the population since doctors started treating people with 'statin' drugs to reduce high blood cholesterol levels.

However, the widespread use of statin drugs has also been shown to reduce the risk of Alzheimer's in many people. In the brain, the deposits of amyloid and the neurofibrillary tangles mentioned earlier in this book (see page 5) may be the results of inflammation caused by excessive deposits of cholesterol, and statins can treat this. In practical terms, all this raises real possibilities of new treatments for Alzheimer's disease, and I look more at statins and at future possible drugs to combat the inflammatory process in Chapter 7, Drug treatments for early dementia (see pages 55–69).

The hormone story

As women may be more susceptible to dementia than men (see page 7), some researchers have connected this with the drop in female sex hormone levels after the menopause. We know that oestrogens act on the brain, because we see oestrogen 'receptors' on the surface of a huge proportion of brain cells. That strongly suggests that oestrogens have widespread effects on all aspects of brain function. One of these effects is to 'upregulate' the brain's acetylcholine system, making it more active. Another is to stimulate the growth of nerve cells that produce acetylcholine. So in theory they should protect doubly against dementia.

At a meeting of Alzheimer Disease International in Helsinki, in 1997, Dr Leon Thal of the University of California, San Diego, spoke of a study of women who had undergone surgical removal of their ovaries without hormone replacement. Even when they were not depressed (a common reaction, understandably, to the operation) they developed some loss of reasoning power. Dr Thal also reported that the women with Alzheimer's disease who responded best to the acetylcholine-raising drug tacrine were those who were also taking hormone replacement therapy (HRT). He suggested that HRT may 'prime' the brain cholinergic cells, so that they will respond better to acetylcholine-raising treatment.

As is the case with anti-inflammatories, long-term HRT does appear to help lower the risk of developing Alzheimer's disease, but the statistics are not as clear or powerful, as they vary greatly from study to study. Dr Thal pointed out that it is difficult to rule out bias in such studies, because HRT tends to be used by women with better education, better access to medical care, and better nutrition than the norm. It is difficult to separate out the effect of HRT from these lifestyle differences, all of which may have played their part in preventing the disease.

The anti-oxidant story

'Anti-oxidants' were all the rage of the health lobby of the 1990s, and look like remaining so through the first years of the twenty-first century. The problem is to prove what they may be doing. The theory is that many diseases result from the effect of 'free oxygen radicals' produced in our tissues by our modern way of eating. Drugs and vitamins that 'scavenge' these oxygen radicals are promoted as reversing or preventing such diseases. They are called anti-oxidants or free radical scavengers. They include vitamins A, C and E, folic acid and beta-carotene.

Fashions for anti-oxidants have included their use against heart disease, diabetes, arthritis, bowel disorders, and a host of other chronic diseases, including cancer, for some of which today's medical treatments have not been satisfactory. Sadly, the anti-oxidants have not lived up to the hopes for them, and sometimes they have proved disastrous.

Take beta-carotene, for example. It was developed because of the belief that carrots are good for you. They contain a lot of beta-carotene, so it was thought to be a good idea to distil out the beta-carotene from them and use it as a food supplement or drug. It was sold in health food shops as a virtual cure-all. Sadly, when it was exposed to properly planned clinical trials the theory did not stand up. In Finland its trial against placebo in 29,000 middle-aged smokers (smoking steeply increases the amounts of free radicals in the tissues – they are blamed for many smoking-related cancers) led to an amazing result. The people who took the 'protective' anti-oxidant had more cancers than those who did not.

This result was followed by the American Physicians Health Study, in which more than 22,000 doctors were given beta-carotene or placebo every day. There was absolutely no health benefit from the beta-carotene. Then the Beta-Carotene and Retinol Efficacy Trial (CARET) was undertaken by the US National Cancer Institute. It followed over 18,000 people at high risk of lung cancer because they smoked or had been exposed to asbestos. CARET had to be stopped early because far more of those taking beta-carotene than taking placebo were developing cancers!

Naturally, dementia has come under the scrutiny of the anti-oxidant lobby. The best evidence that anti-oxidants might help in Alzheimer's disease comes from Dr Thal's report in Helsinki. The study he presented showed that a combination of selegiline (an anti-depressant drug) and vitamin E (alpha-tocopherol) delayed entry into nursing homes and slowed down deterioration in the ability to live normally at home. There was no effect on cognition. Although vitamin E had a relatively slight effect, Dr Thal felt that any progress towards keeping people longer at home was worthwhile.

So far there is no evidence that other anti-oxidants have any effect on established dementia. Very large-scale trials will be needed to prove any effect, either way – and there is very little incentive to do them. In the meantime it seems that if anti-oxidants do have any effect at all, it is best to wrap them up as nature intended – to eat plenty of fruit and vegetables, and not take them as vitamin or artificial dietary supplements.

Images of the brain in Alzheimer's

We have dealt so far in this chapter with the work of the geneticists and the biochemists but the really startling work has been done by the experts in brain imaging. I was privileged to take the official notes at a meeting in Heidelberg on the subject. I was astonished then to learn that the experts in this field can take brain cells during surgery from people (say, from tumour or stroke patients) and keep them alive in cultures, in which they can be studied as individual cells.

Cultured brain cells can be exposed to all sorts of nutrients and damage to see how they react, and cells from different regions of the brain, from people of different ages, and with no dementia or in different stages of dementia, can be studied. Such work has produced amazing new knowledge of how brain cells work, and which part of the brain is responsible for which function. In particular, studies like this, along with new techniques to make images of the brain in living people, have hugely increased our knowledge of the processes that lead to dementia.

Most importantly, these new imaging techniques can be used to make the diagnosis of dementia, and to divide it into subtypes, and to follow accurately its progress. Eventually, when we develop more effective treatments, they should be able to follow the improvements they produce.

Today, the two main brain imaging techniques are computer-assisted tomography (commonly known as CT scans) and magnetic resonance imaging (MRI). CT detects changes in the brain such as tumours, hydrocephalus (increased fluid pressure within the brain), severely reduced circulation to the brain (such as after a stroke), and severe atrophy (shrinkage) of the brain substance. However, it is not good at detailing the small changes that might be seen in Alzheimer's.

MRI is more sensitive than CT in detecting the changes in Alzheimer's and other forms of dementia. It can pick up specific changes in the parts of the brain surface and of sites within the brain that are affected by Alzheimer's. MRI has the advantage that it can be used to measure the volume of structures in the brain that are known to be affected early and preferentially in Alzheimer's. Shrinkage of these structures (which are to do with gathering and retaining memory) is linked with dementia, but has to be differentiated from the normal shrinkage that occurs with ageing. MRI is continually being refined to give more precise images of the brain.

The real breakthrough in brain imaging, however, has come with two newer techniques, positron emission tomography (PET) and single proton emission computed tomography (SPECT). They can actually measure what the brain is doing. For example, they show the active circulation within the brain in detail. They show changes in the metabolism of the brain tissues – which parts of the brain are working healthily and which are not. They can even map the 'receptors' on nerve cell surfaces, so that they can tell the physician which cells are receptive, for example, to acetylcholine or oestrogen, and whether the neurotransmitter systems are working normally or not.

CT and MRI scans are now routine hospital procedures. PET and SPECT are still mainly research tools, but will surely be in much more common use within the next few years, especially for the diagnosis and follow-up of Alzheimer's.

It must be said here that dementia is a diagnosis made in the clinic and is based on the patient's symptoms and history and their subsequent development. It is not made solely from the results of CT, MRI, PET or SPECT scans. Nor is it made from the study of the electrical currents within the brain – electro-encephalography, or EEG. There are EEG changes typical of dementia, but they, too, must be considered along with all the other findings, and do not make the diagnosis on their own. All these techniques are used to confirm, or judge the extent of, or follow the progress of, dementia that is already strongly suspected by the doctor. Or they are used to rule out or identify other conditions in the brain that may mimic dementias, such as a stroke or clot, multiple minor strokes, hydrocephalus, a tumour or abscess.

The reservations expressed in the last paragraph, however, should not belittle what techniques like CT, MRI, PET, SPECT and EEG have done to improve our understanding of the brain, how it works, and what happens when it goes wrong. For example, they have shown beyond doubt that Alzheimer's disease is not just a matter of accelerated ageing. In fact, it is completely unlike the ageing process. Different parts of the brain are affected by Alzheimer's and the normal ageing process, and the changes in them with age differs, too.

The changes in Alzheimer's affect the parts of the brain specifically responsible for learning, memory and reasoning. They are shown in Figure 2.2. The brain is often compared to a computer, with a centre for collecting inputs (from the eyes, ears, tongue, nose, skin), from which there are outflow tracks to storage centres to put the data in memory banks. There are also tracks from the input collecting centres and memory centres to centres for reasoning and calculation. And of course there is consciousness. Where that is centred is more difficult to understand, but studies of conditions in which consciousness is lost (such as under anaesthesia or coma states) suggest that it is the result of a network of interconnections throughout the brain surface. Brain imaging techniques have convinced researchers to change their ideas of how the brain works. It is more like a network of computers, with multiple interconnections, than a single computer working from a floppy disc (the input centre) and transferring the new data every so often to the hard disc (the memory centre). Put as simply as possible, the incoming messages from our five senses are gathered into our hippocampus during the daytime. The hippocampus sits in the centre of the brain. When we fall asleep, all the data collected that day is transferred by way of long neurofibrils to cells in the rest of the brain – some to the front, some to the sides, and some to the base of the front of the brain. Figure 2.2 shows where these areas are.

What the brain imaging systems, along with EEG and postmortem and operation specimen findings, have shown is that Alzheimer's affects all these areas of gathering and retaining memory, and the parts of the brain that give us our ability to make sense of the new data.

The area that seems to be affected first is the hippocampus. In early Alzheimer's hippocampal cells shaped like pyramids – so naturally they are called pyramidal cells – die off first. As they are the cells that receive the incoming data from our senses, the change affects the ability to remember what has been happening that day. As the hippocampal cells die off, and the tangles and amyloid plaques appear, the hippocampus itself shrinks, and that shrinkage is obvious on brain scans. A shrunken hippocampus is one sign of progressive dementia.

As the disease progresses, the same changes occur in the surface cells of the brain – the cerebral cortex. That leads to loss of longer-term memory and the ability to understand everyday things and to make reasoned judgements. PET studies show that the acetylcholine-secreting nerve cells are the first to go, and that even when the disease is advancing they are still lost in preference to other cells.

Robert D. Terry, of the University of California, has studied the changes in the brain over many years in people ageing normally and in those with Alzheimer's. He found that the brain loses weight steadily throughout life, mainly due to loss of the largest brain cells. However, in the Alzheimer's brain the rate of weight loss is much steeper.

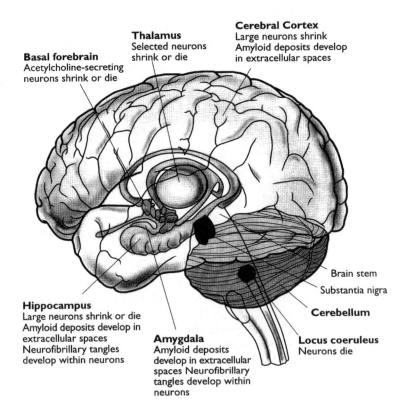

Thalamus
Selected neurons
shrink or die

Cerebral Cortex
Large neurons shrink
Amyloid deposits develop
in extracellular spaces

Basal forebrain
Acetylcholine-secreting
neurons shrink or die

Brain stem

Substantia nigra

Cerebellum

Hippocampus
Large neurons shrink or die
Amyloid deposits develop in
extracellular spaces
Neurofibrillary tangles
develop within neurons

Amygdala
Amyloid deposits
develop in extracellular
spaces Neurofibrillary
tangles develop within
neurons

Locus coeruleus
Neurons die

Figure 2.2 Brain structures involved in learning, memory and reasoning

Some brain image experts say they can verify the diagnosis of Alzheimer's from the MRI finding that specific parts of the brain, such as the hippocampus, the amygdala and the temporal lobe of the cerebral cortex (see Figure 2.2), have shrunk. Others say that such shrinkage is common in normal ageing. This is where PET and SPECT come into their own. When they show that the blood flow through these same areas, particularly in the temporal lobe, is abnormal, along with the MRI changes in volume, this is a strong indication of Alzheimer's.

The EEG in Alzheimer's

Electro-encephalographs have a popular image of being extremely scientific: films in which the hero has a brain problem – including Frankenstein's monster – usually include them being wired up to an EEG. The experts have a brief look at all the squiggles on the roll of paper and make an instant diagnosis.

Real life isn't like that. There are changes in the EEG in dementia, but they are difficult to assess and not particularly informative. A new science of quantitative EEG assessment, using computer analysis, is beginning to solve these problems, but there is still no agreement among the experts about which changes truly reflect Alzheimer's disease, at least when the EEG is taken while the patient is awake. There is more agreement about the EEG changes in dementia when the person is asleep, and as they appear early in the illness, they may even be used in future to make an early diagnosis. So a sleeping EEG may form part of the future routine diagnostic process in people suspected of having dementia.

Future biochemical tests?

For most diseases there are simple blood tests that can confirm the diagnosis. Among the simplest perhaps is a low haemoglobin level or red cell count in anaemia, or a high blood glucose level in diabetes, or a high urea level in kidney disease, or a high white cell count in an infection.

It would be very helpful if there were a similar test for dementia but so far we are still searching for one. Two such tests show some promise. One is the level of a subtance called Tau protein in the fluid

21

around the spinal cord – the cerebrospinal fluid (CSF). It is raised well above normal levels even in the early stages of Alzheimer's dementia, and it may relate to amyloid deposits or tangles in the brain. However, the current methods of measuring it are too unreliable for routine use, and it would be unacceptable to put every person suspected of having Alzheimer's through the ordeal of a spinal 'tap'. We need a reliable blood test.

A future test may come from work on a substance called melanotransferin, or P97. P97 is believed to control the amounts of iron passing into cells. Its levels in blood are higher than normal in people with Alzheimer's and continue to rise as the disease worsens. So it may help initially to give a diagnosis and then, on repeated blood tests, to follow the progress of the disease.

Finally, there is an odd test that may be available to general practitioners if its reliability is confirmed. L.C.M. Scinto reported in *Science* the use of simple eye drops as a marker of Alzheimer's disease. When he dropped the pupil-dilating drug tropicamide into the eye of a patient with Alzheimer's disease, the pupil opened up to its maximum dilation much faster than normal. The test fulfilled all the criteria for a good diagnostic system – it was fast, simple, cheap and reliable. It was accurate in 94 out of every 100 Alzheimer's patients. It hasn't been universally adopted yet, but some doctors find it useful.

Misunderstandings about dementia

This chapter would not be complete without listing the things that are popularly thought to cause dementia, but that in fact do not. For example, it is not caused by 'hardening of the arteries', which is a normal stiffening of the blood vessel walls that occurs with age. Most 'hardened' arteries take enough blood to the brain to maintain the circulation there, and in any case, Alzheimer's disease is a primary affliction of the brain cells, and not of the circulation that takes blood to them.

Dementia is NOT caused by either under-use or over-use of the brain. Many studies, it is true, have found it to be more common in people who have had fewer years of full-time education than in people graduating from universities, but that may simply be due to the fact that better educated people can hide their dementia for longer. They may be able to cope better than the less educated with the loss of much of their reasoning power and memory, perhaps hiding their loss under a more self-confident mental veneer.

Powerful sources of stress, such as bereavement, retirement or moving house, do not cause dementia, but they may bring a previously hidden dementia out into the open. The loss of a lifelong partner, who may have been protecting a patient from the outside world, is a classic time for the neighbours and family to learn that something is badly wrong but it has usually been going on for years. The same goes for the loss of the usual routine that comes with retirement and moving home. The mildly demented person can usually cope if he or she is following a strict, unchanging routine. When that changes, confusion follows, and the true state of the mental loss is at last appreciated by family and friends.

The other scares have been environmental – the most publicized being the aluminium one. That comes from the finding of excess amounts of aluminium in the brains of people with dementia. Of course, finding a relationship between aluminium and dementia does not prove that the first causes the second. No-one could disprove, for example, that the dementia may have come first and that the brain abnormality allowed a higher than normal amount of aluminium to enter it. In any case, the aluminium theory has been abandoned since a large study of the brains of people dying from Alzheimer's found normal aluminium levels in them. There is plenty of aluminium in tea, anti-perspirants and in antacid medicines, yet high use of any of these has never been linked to Alzheimer's.

Massive overdoses of aluminium, however, may be a different matter. On 6 July 1988, twenty tonnes of aluminium sulphate were accidentally tipped into a water reservoir used by the 20,000 people living in and around Camelford in Cornwall. Many became acutely ill, with rashes, indigestion, muscle aches and pains, general malaise and lack of concentration and short-term memory problems. Two years later 400 people still had after-effects. Three years later 55 people were considering litigation against the water company for chronic illnesses allegedly linked to the contamination. They were largely dismissed as being due to anxiety.

That view has been revised. Paul Altmann and colleagues re-examined these 55 people and 15 siblings close in age to them who had not been exposed to the aluminium. They found that the people who had been exposed had lower intelligence than expected from their previous tests and their relatives' performances, and that they scored unexpectedly poorly on specialized tests of reactions to visual stimuli. In other words, their intellect had been significantly damaged by their exposure to aluminium.

This is not to say that aluminium has anything to do with the usual forms of dementia, but it suggests that it may play a part in some cases. We are going to hear a lot more about the Camelford people in the future.

Nor does it seem that Alzheimer's disease is caused by other poisons in the environment. Links have been suggested, for example, between Alzheimer's and long-term exposure to lead or to agricultural chemicals, like the organo-phosphates used in sheep dips. They are indeed poisonous to nerve tissues, but they lead to very particular symptoms and mental problems that are quite different from Alzheimer's, and they are mostly reversible on stopping the contact with them. The relationship between abnormal mental problems and lead has been known for hundreds of years. That's why Lewis Carroll chose a hatter to be mad at Alice's tea party. Hatters used lead to stiffen and preserve top hats and were badly affected by it. 'Madness' was a common end for them. But their symptoms were not the same as those of people with dementia. And the pesticide problem usually affects the peripheral nerves, with weakness and abnormal feelings in the limbs, rather than mental illness.

Nor is dementia just an extreme form of old age: 80 per cent of people over 75 years old continue to think normally and enjoy a normal intellectual life. They may forget things from time to time, but they retain all they need to enjoy a good social life and to look after themselves well. Alzheimer's and the other forms of dementia are definitely illnesses, and not just an extreme example of ageing. The changes in the brain in Alzheimer's and in the other forms of dementia are clearly different from ageing, and are disease processes, not just the result of mental 'wear and tear'. They should always be treated as such.

What Alzheimer's probably IS

I can find no better person to guide me on what Alzheimer's IS than my colleague Zaven Khachaturian. Drawing a recent meeting on Alzheimer's to a close, he summarized the current research into the disease as follows:

There are 3,000 scientists working on the ageing brain. In the United States, 28 centres are carrying out longitudinal studies of subjects available for clinical trials, and they will soon have clinical data on 30,000 patients, to be used for further research. [Similar research is ongoing in Europe.]

Before the 1970s there were no clues on the causes of, or changes in, the disease. Then British discoveries that there were biochemical deficits in the disease brought research biochemists into the field. Risk factors leading to Alzheimer's, such as brain injuries and the ApoE gene, also gave clues for developing treatment. Neurotransmitter deficits in cholinergic and other messenger systems in the brain have been identified and are targets for research.

PET has identified metabolic deficiencies in the use of glucose in the brain in Alzheimer's, and they are also a target for treatment, as are other biochemical abnormalities. The plaques and tangles are under intense study, and much more is known about their chemistry than before. The loss of intellect and skills is largely due to the loss of synapses [the connections between brain cells] and much more is known about this process.

Three inter-related systems maintain the viability of brain cells:

- Circulation. Lack of circulation leads to death of brain cells after strokes. However, abnormalities in the smallest vessels may deprive brain cells of oxygen and nutrition without there being any symptom of stroke.
- Ability to communicate. The sole purpose of brain nerve cells is to communicate. They use various chemical signals (neuro-transmitters, peptides, growth promoters and 'neurotrophics') to do so. There are also messenger systems within the cells that regulate gene activity – all these systems may be altered in Alzheimer's.
- Ability to self-repair. We are born with enough nerve cells to do us far more than a lifetime. However, each nerve cell is constantly repairing its surfaces and its ability to make proteins. This self-repair system is broken down in Alzheimer's, which is why the tangles and amyloid plaques form and the cells die prematurely. Understanding of how this happens will lead to new treatments.

When the research projects will bear fruit is not easy to predict, but there is huge pressure on the researchers to succeed. The world's population of over-65s will rise from 390 million at the time of writing to 800 million by 2025, reaching 10 per cent of the total population. One in four of them will eventually develop dementia. It is a time bomb which we must stop ticking. However, Professor Ian Hindmarch, of the University of Surrey, is among medical experts who remain optimistic. There are already active drugs against dementia, and others must follow.

3

Diagnosing a possible case

There are many reasons to make the diagnosis of dementia as early as possible. The first and foremost is because many people who seem to have it actually don't. As mentioned in Chapter 1, other physical illnesses, like thyroid disease, can mimic dementia, and this can easily be reversed by giving the thyroid hormone thyroxine by mouth just once a day. The patient may be depressed, rather than demented, and depression can respond very well to modern drugs plus psychological and social support to reverse or remove its cause.

The second reason for making an early diagnosis is so that treatment can start as soon as possible. That involves not only drugs to delay its progress, but also all the ways in which the life of both the patient and the carer can be improved and planned. This will be described in the following chapters.

So the first priority is to investigate a possible new case of dementia very thoroughly. Only when all reversible causes have been ruled out, and/or brain imaging changes (see Chapter 2) are typical of dementia, should the diagnosis be made.

Obviously there are some people who, at the first medical appointment, are so typical in their story and symptoms, that the doctor has little doubt. But even they can be deceptive, so it is incumbent on the doctor to put everyone through the diagnostic mill. That involves a lot of questions about the person's family life, as well as about their current problems. And it means a detailed physical examination, with necessary blood tests for laboratory analysis. After that, there are measures of memory, mood, intelligence and social activities to be made that not only confirm or reject the diagnosis, but also pinpoint the stage it has reached.

Let's take three typical case histories to show how the diagnostic 'ladder' works in practice.

David: David is a 69-year-old retired accountant who was never ill. His last visit to the doctor was for holiday vaccinations three years before. Nothing untoward had been noted then. His wife had brought him this time because he had been restless and anxious lately. He no longer bothered to watch television. He found it difficult to fill in his cheques – a big change for an accountant. He couldn't remember where he put personal things, like his glasses or slippers. He constantly had to ask his wife where they were. He found it difficult to keep up a conversation, often forgetting what had been said a few minutes before. This would make him unreasonably angry, a new experience for his wife, who said that he had always been a placid and reasonable man. Yet he was neat and tidy as ever, washed and dressed scrupulously, and could keep up appearances in company outside the home, so that few of his friends had an inkling of his real plight.

Oh, and one other thing, his wife added, as an afterthought. David was not sleeping well. He was getting to sleep all right in the evening, but had started wakening very early each morning, often around 4 or 5 o'clock, and couldn't drop off again, no matter how hard he tried.

John: John is 72, a retired engineer. His wife, who brought him in, was worried because all he did was sit and sleep through the daytime, yet he still managed to sleep well at night. She noticed that he hardly moved, rarely took part in conversation, and certainly did not initiate it. When he did move he was slow and deliberate. He was no longer interested in the paper: previously an avid reader, he had given up his daily crossword some months before. His wife thought that his features had coarsened recently, his skin becoming thicker, and he had lost a lot of hair. She was curious about this, because he had had a good head of hair until a year ago. She asked if this was not an unusually late stage of life to start going bald.

Megan: Megan, a retired journalist, is 75. She came herself to the doctor because she was finding it difficult to remember everyday words. She had taken to writing down things to do, such as housework, bill paying and shopping, because she was forgetting them. Now she was forgetting where she was putting her lists. However, she was still singing in her church choir, though she had had to give up her drama club because she could no longer learn lines. One other admission from her was that she was much more easily tired than before. She put all these problems down to her advancing age, and thought she might need a 'tonic'.

Their doctors followed the same diagnostic pathway in each case and came up with very different answers.

David's problem

When his doctor started to ask David questions, he was fairly sure, from the story told by his wife, that he was dealing with a case of dementia. However, the answers to the questions led him in another direction. David had taken to retirement very badly: he had lived for his work, and now he felt useless and worthless. He saw nothing but deterioration into old age in front of him, and (in his wife's absence) admitted to misery at the thought of spending it with a partner whose company he could no longer bear. Mental tests showed that he still had a good brain, both for reasoning and for memory, but he scored very high on a 'depression scale' questionnaire.

David's underlying problem is severe depression. His treatment is going to be long and complex, a combination of anti-depressant drugs and psychotherapy, including even at this late age counselling on the marriage. He and his wife have a difficult road ahead, but at least it is not going to be complicated by dementia.

Depression can easily cause forgetfulness, anxiety, changes in mood, especially anger. And a strong pointer to it in his case was the sleep disturbance. Early morning wakening is a classic sign of depression – it is not particularly a problem in early dementia.

Although the diagnosis of depression was clear, David was also subjected to the routine battery of blood tests for his general physical health. He got the all-clear for liver and kidney and heart function and also for thyroid gland function. It was considered there was no need for brain imaging tests, unless he did not respond to treatment.

John's problem

John also did not have dementia. He was a walking textbook case of myxoedema – a thyroid gland that had given up. The thyroid gland in the neck is the body's accelerator. Its hormone, thyroxine, speeds up the rate at which the body turns over energy. So everything gets faster – the heartbeat, the rate at which we think, how fast we move and react to stimuli. When we lose our ability to produce thyroxine we slow down to the basic level. Everything slows down: the heart beats around 60 times a minute or less, we think more slowly, we react more slowly, we couldn't get up to a run even in an emergency. Mentally and emotionally we shut down. We lose the hair on top of our heads (and sometimes grow it more on our face if we are female), and the skin coarsens as the circulation through it slows and the skin cells shed much more slowly.

In fact, his doctor made the diagnosis of John's case almost as he walked through the door but he confirmed it with a blood thyroxine test. He was secreting almost none at all. After just one tablet of thyroxine John started to feel better and act faster. Within two weeks he was back to his old self and even beginning to grow his hair again. He will need the tablets, once a day, for the rest of his life.

However, even though the diagnosis was obvious, John was put through the same mental and memory tests as David. He scored low on the mental tests and on the memory tests, but largely because he was so slow in performing them. When asked to take them again three weeks later, he performed well on both.

John's other blood tests showed no other organ abnormality, so that he was given a physical all-clear. His very good response to thyroxine convinced his doctor that there was no need to order further tests, such as brain imaging.

Megan's problem

Sadly, the outlook is not so good for Megan. Although she was the only one of the three who had presented herself to the doctor, she was the one with Alzheimer's. The mixture of forgetfulness and absent-mindedness, excessive tiredness, difficulty in remembering common words, inability to learn new things, and withdrawing from her usual social network (like the drama club) filled her doctor with foreboding.

It was confirmed by the results of tests of her mental state. She had difficulty in recalling words, names and numbers said to her a few minutes before, could not name objects from pictures of them, had difficulty copying simple geometric figures and in constructing elementary toy building block structures. All these tests had been passed with ease by David and by John, once he had started on his thyroxine.

In short, she had much more wrong with her memory, reasoning powers, and mechanical and artistic abilities than her original interview had suggested. Nevertheless, she was friendly and co-operative, was well dressed and clean, and was not in the least depressed or in any way obviously mentally abnormal. All she asked for was her 'tonic' to make her feel better.

Where was her doctor to go from here? A widow, she lived with her 73-year-old sister, also a widow, whom her doctor knows to be in good health. So he could assume there would be good home support. The second action was to explain that she needed further tests before a diagnosis could be made, and that it might be a good idea for her to bring her sister along so that they could be explained. The third action was to make an appointment with the local specialist in Alzheimer's, to arrange for a more detailed assessment of possible dementia. This will probably include the brain imaging tests described in Chapter 2.

Her doctor is fairly sure that they will confirm Alzheimer's, but there is still the remote possibility of a focal brain problem, like an abscess, tumour or old clot from an unrecognized stroke or forgotten injury. Although the history, symptoms and signs do not fit any of these diagnoses, it is only fair to look for them. She must have her chance to rule out a treatable condition before the long journey into Alzheimer's begins. Her sister, too, must have that chance, because she will be living every day with her.

If the specialist diagnoses Megan as having Alzheimer's, then she and her sister need to know what is likely to lie ahead, and how they can best be helped. This is the subject of the next few chapters.

4

Specialist tests for diagnosis

Megan has gone to her general practitioner to sort out why she has become forgetful and confused. Reversible causes, like depression or thyroid underactivity, or a possible brain lesion like a tumour, abscess or clot, have been ruled out. What happens next?

We now have to find out the extent of the confusion and forgetfulness, and perhaps loss of reasoning power. That is best done using a series of mental tests devised especially for dementia. There are a host of them, and they all take longer to complete than the usual general practitioner's consulting time. That's why an appointment is usually made for a 'memory assessment clinic' in your local district general hospital. The first memory assessment clinics specifically for older people were set up in most countries in the late 1970s, but it was only in the 1990s that their importance was recognized, and such clinics became as routine as, say, hearing assessment and eye clinics.

Memory assessment is not a painful or frightening experience. In some versions you are seated comfortably at a table, and asked to complete simple tasks either with pencil and paper, or at a simple computer keyboard. In others you sit in an easy chair, and have a conversation with the tester, who will ask you everyday questions, and note down the answers. The tests are usually carried out by a nurse trained in memory assessment, in a friendly, relaxed environment: there are no white-coated doctors or fierce-looking instruments to overawe you.

The most commonly used of these tests is the 'Mini Mental State Examination' or MMSE. It asks a series of questions, and gives numbers to the answers, so that an all-correct score is 30. It is usually assumed that a score of 26 or more is normal, although highly educated people may score in the upper 20s and still have early Alzheimer's disease. A simple user-friendly MMSE is given here:

Question	Score
What is the day of the week?	1
What is the month?	1
What is the date?	1
What is the season?	1
What is the year?	1
What city/town are we in?	1
What is the county?	1
What is the country?	1
What building are we in?	1
What floor are we on?	1
Repeat after me 'ball car man' (don't score)	
Repeat again 'ball car man' (score after second trial)	3
Spell the word WORLD (don't score)	
Now try to spell it backwards (DLROW) (score)	5
What were the three words you were asked to remember?	3
What is this called? (show a watch)	1
What is this called? (show a pencil)	1
Repeat after me 'no ifs and buts'	1
Read and do what is written down (card bears the sentence 'close your eyes')	1
Write a short sentence	1
Copy this drawing (two interlocking pentagons)	1
Take this paper in your left hand (right hand if person is left-handed)	1
Fold it in half	1
Put it on the floor	1
Total score	**30**

Taken all together, the answers to these questions form a simple guide to a person's reasoning power ('cognition'), sense of time and place ('orientation'), memory, attention, comprehension, naming ability, and practical skills, all of which can be faulty in early Alzheimer's. However, MMSE has its problems.

One is that the research team who developed it never meant it to become the main means of making the diagnosis of Alzheimer's disease or other forms of dementia. It was designed to be a fast, simple screening test that would help researchers choose subjects for trials of treatment of dementia. People who scored between 10 and 26 were chosen for studies, because it was assumed that any worthwhile treatment might improve the scores enough for the numbers to be put through a statistical analysis. People who scored below 10 were assumed to be too far along the disease process to be treatable. People scoring above 26 probably did not have dementia, or any improvement in them might not be measurable on MMSE. If they did have very early dementia, any deterioration might be too slow for an advantage of treatment to be measurable, at least on the MMSE.

But there is a stronger objection to using MMSE alone either to diagnose or to assess the severity of dementia. Many people don't like to be subjected to MMSE. They feel that being questioned in this way has an underlying purpose that is perhaps not in their interest, so they don't co-operate. At the 9th Alzheimer Europe Meeting in London in July 1999, Margaret Anne Tibbs, of the Alzheimer's Society, reported on a study by the Bradford Dementia Group. Of 100 people in ten residential homes for the elderly with MMSE scores below 20, a third scored zero. Yet from simply watching them in their normal daily routine, their memory, cognition, understanding, orientation and co-ordination should have produced far higher scores. They had effectively withdrawn their consent to be tested, by not co-operating with the testers.

Mrs Tibbs also stressed that some of the MMSE questions are irrelevant to many elderly people: they don't need to know the day and date, or the county they are living in, so why should they bother about them? A better test is whether they know their way about the home in which they are living, and whether they recognize or know the people they are living with.

MMSE is not even an accurate indicator of whether or not a person has dementia. At the same Alzheimer Europe meeting, Nia White, of the University of Wales, described the consequences of asking general practitioners to use MMSE in their annual screening of all their (apparently normal) patients over 75 years old. On the basis of the MMSE scores, 237 of 606 people were asked to take part in a second test, the Geriatric Mental State Examination (GMS), which is a more detailed and accurate assessment of dementia, but takes much longer to perform. Of the 237, 148 were found to be normal, with no dementia; 65 refused to take part in GMS; and only 24 turned out to have dementia. The normal results tended to be in the younger over-75s: older people with lower MMSEs were more likely to refuse further tests. So it seems that the more vulnerable people are to dementia, the less likely they are to co-operate with testing to prove their disability.

This isn't surprising. Suspicion of other people and their motives is part of early dementia, and an underlying reason for lack of co-operation. And with dementia come other mental problems, such as disturbed and abnormal thoughts and behaviour. They need assessment, too, because they cause great distress to both dementia sufferers and their carers. They are also amenable to modern treatments.

So the researchers have developed a host of rating scales by which dementia in all its aspects can be diagnosed, even without the patient's co-operation, and which can then be used to follow the progress of the disease, for better or for worse. They are described briefly below. Most measure similar aspects of dementia, but they differ in detail, depending on the country in which they were designed and tested, and often on the particular interests of the research teams developing them.

These tests fall into five groups:

1 Tests of the patients' cognition that need their co-operation, like MMSE.
2 Doctor's assessments of the severity of dementia from observing the patients, or 'global' assessments.
3 Global assessments of changes in dementia, which can differ from the above tests.
4 Ratings of behaviour patterns.
5 Assessments of how well patients are coping with daily life, or 'activities of daily living' (ADL) scales.

This is not the place to describe every dementia assessment scale in detail. There are so many of them, and they are becoming so complex, that they would need another book of this size to do them justice. But every person with dementia will at some time be faced with one or another of them, so here are a few of the more widely used ones.

Cognitive tests

MMSE has been described above. A test along the same lines, but much more detailed, is the Alzheimer's Assessment Scale cognitive subscale (ADAS-cog). It is now the accepted way to measure change in Alzheimer's disease in the clinical trials of new drugs. There are ADAS-cog versions in French, German, Italian, Spanish, Finnish, Danish, Greek, Hebrew and Japanese, so that trials of drugs in many countries can compare like-for-like. The United States National Institute of Aging Alzheimer Disease Cooperative Study group has been expanding it, so that it covers the patient's attention and 'executive' abilities (ability to plan and perform co-ordinated actions).

ADAS-cog is a battery of brief tests, including word recall, naming objects, understanding and carrying out commands, constructing and forming ideas, orientation in time and place, word recognition, speaking and understanding language, and recall of previous instructions. It takes an hour to complete and scores are marked on the numbers of errors made – from nil to 70.

ADAS-cog is the gold standard, but it needs a very patient questioner and an extremely co-operative patient with a good attention span. So it is mainly used for trials of drugs, where it is essential to be able to measure subtle changes in the progression of the disease, either for the worse or better. Interestingly, it is accurate enough to show differences between the newer drugs and placebo in large trials in patients with early Alzheimer's disease.

In routine memory clinics, where time is at a premium, patients are not in trials, and there is a need simply for practical assessment of the patient's illness and progress, shorter tests, on similar lines to ADAS-cog, are used. One is the Information-Concentration-Memory (ICM) test. It consists of 27 questions assessing orientation, long-term memory, recall, concentration and performance. It takes 20 to 30 minutes.

The Syndrom Kurztest (SKT) is used mainly in German-speaking countries. It consists of nine performance subtests, limited to one minute each, including naming objects and numerals, immediate and delayed recall, arranging and replacing blocks, and counting symbols. The score depends on the time people take to complete it, so that they have to be fast to score well. SKT takes under 15 minutes.

As the disease progresses, or in some dementias in which progress to a late stage is faster than usual, the Severe Impairment Battery (SIB) may be used. SIB is for people who score 10 or below on

MMSE. It uses questions needing only one-word answers or one-step commands to be understood and obeyed, and assesses social behaviour, memory, orientation, language, attention, mechanical abilities, and co-ordination of visual and physical abilities.

Global rating scales

All the above cognitive tests need the patient's co-operation. To add to them, or if the patient is unwilling or unable to co-operate, the clinicians' global impressions are used. Different countries, indeed almost all individual dementia specialists, have adopted scales best suited to themselves, so that it would be pointless listing them all. They all use a system in which questions are asked of the doctors and carers who see the patient from day to day, as well as of the patients themselves.

In the Clinical Dementia Rating Scale (CDR) the tester uses worksheets to conduct a structured interview with both patient and carer: it assesses cognition, daily practical living and social relationships. It entails scoring six sections, so that the final score ranges from 0 (normal) to 18 (very severe dementia).

The Global Deterioration Scale (GDS), devised by Professor Barry Reisburg of New York, rates seven stages of dementia, and assesses the progression of the disease cognitively, physically and according to behaviour. Roughly, a GDS grade of 1 is normal, of 3 is early dementia (or as Professor Reisburg would put it, incipient dementia or late confusion), 5 is middle dementia, and 7 late dementia. GDS is assessed by a doctor with access to all sources of information about the patient. Because it graphically describes the progress of dementia from its early beginnings, it is described in much more detail in the next chapter.

Not everyone agrees with the detailed GDS system: many think it is too rigid or too complicated. The Sandoz Clinical Assessment Geriatric Scale – or SCAG – is often used instead. It stresses what are considered to be 18 cardinal signs and symptoms of dementia, relatively ignoring the changes in mood, behaviour, and the ability to cope with the everyday practicalities of life.

Scales like these do give clues to doctors and carers on how people with dementia may be managed, and perhaps indicate what lies in the immediate future. For example, CDR tests of hundreds of people with dementia showed that if they have delusions and hallucinations in the early stages (CDR of 1) they are more likely to deteriorate faster than people at a similar stage without them.

The problem with all these cases remains that people with Alzheimer's disease vary widely, and a rating on one scale may be very different from that on another. And when they are used to measure the effects of drugs on the disease, it is difficult to relate changes in global test scores to real improvement that matters in the family environment. This is why Global change scores were introduced.

Global change scores

Like all the other tests, global change scores are abbreviated into collections of capital letters. They may seem forbidding to people unused to medical measurement, but the acronyms are convenient for medical journals so I have reproduced them here. Doctors use them, in the form of a brief but structured interview, to see the effect of a treatment.

The most commonly used global change score is the Clinical Global Impression (CGI). It was used in depression, anxiety and schizophrenia before being applied to dementia, so that it has been very fully evaluated. It consists of 7-point ratings of severity and change, and produces an index of efficacy that contrasts the change for the better or worse with any side-effects of treatment.

CGI depends on doctors using it being skilled enough to draw the appropriate conclusions and to assess meaningful changes. It asks them to choose a response to treatment ranging from 1 – very much improved, 2 – much improved, 3 – minimally improved, 4 – not changed, 5 – minimally worse, 6 – much worse, and 7 – very much worse. This type of assessment is obviously subjective, but it remains the basis of all the other global scales of measurement of change in dementia.

The United States Food and Drugs Administration (FDA) modified the CGI into the FDA Clinicians' Interview-Based Impression of Change (CIBIC). This was intended to be based entirely on information collected by the doctor from the patient alone without input from carers or any other third parties. It keeps the CGI 7-point scale. Other groups have modified the CGI score further: they include the ADCS-CGIC score, developed by the American National Institute of Aging for its Alzheimer's Disease Cooperative Study (ADCS). This asks the doctor to examine 15 areas of cognition, behaviour, and social and daily activities. New York University and Novartis Pharmaceuticals together have produced the NYU CIBIC+ scale which involves both patient and caregiver in a half-structured interview.

The idea behind all these global change scales is that they will identify a change large enough to be meaningful in that they may show how treatment can really improve the quality of life for dementia sufferers. However, they remain imprecise and do not address what is often the major problem for carers and sufferers alike – the psychiatric symptoms that go along with dementia. For that scales that measure behaviour and daily living activities are needed.

Behavioural scales

Sadly, the loss of intellect and understanding are not the only symptoms of dementia. Dementia also brings with it delusions, hallucinations, agitation, anxiety, aggression and depression. Very often it is these symptoms, and not the dementia, that finally leads to a family's decision not to continue to look after their relative at home. Treatments aimed at them are at least as important as those directed at the dementia itself.

Unfortunately many drugs trials deliberately do not enter patients with problem behaviour and psychiatric symptoms, because they naturally have a high drop-out rate. It is only recently that the researchers have realized that drugs that improve behaviour, rather than intellect, are probably most welcome to the family of disturbed patients. Scales have at last been devised to measure such effects.

Probably the most commonly used is the ADAS-non-cognitive subscale (ADAS-noncog). It assesses tearfulness, depression, concentration, uncooperativeness, delusions, hallucinations, pacing (walking about aimlessly), physical activity, tremors, and appetite. Each subsection carries a scale of 0 to 5, and scores range from 0 to 50 (the most severe). ADAS-noncog is often combined with ADAS-cog for a total ADAS score. It is usually rated by the tester in a meeting with the patient.

The Behaviour Rating Scale for Dementia of the Consortium to Establish a Registry for Alzheimer's Disease (CERAD BRSD) is based on an interview with the carers, and notes the frequency of depressive symptoms, psychotic symptoms, poor self-control, irritability/aggression, introversion, apathy, and mood swings. Similar scales are the Behavioural Pathology in AD scale (BEHAVE-AD), the Brief Psychiatric Rating Scale (BPRS), the Neuropsychiatric Inventory (NPI), and the Cohen-Mansfield Agitation Inventory (CMAI), the last being designed for nurses to give.

Functional scales

The people who best know how dementia affects patients in a practical way, such as their abilities to cope with the usual routine of daily life, are their carers and relatives. Functional scales have been devised to measure the effects of dementia.

Historically, the two most used functional scales have been the Physical Self-Maintenance Scale (PSMS) and the Instrumental Activities of Daily Living (IADL) scale. IADL assesses performance in telephoning, shopping, food preparation, housekeeping, laundry, use of transport, finances and responsibility for medicines. It is rated by the caregiver, and its scores range from 4 to 30 points. PSMS assesses toilet manners, feeding, dressing, grooming, washing and bathing and ability to get around. It is rated by a trained 'rater' on information given by the caregiver, and scores range from 6 to 30 points.

PSMS and IADL have recently been superseded by scales that expand on each of these areas of concern, and that remove gender bias (many older men have never been good in the kitchen, for example, while many older women have traditionally left their management of finances to their men). They include the Progressive Deterioration Scale (PDS) and the Interview for Deterioration in Daily living activities in Dementia (IDDD).

In the Disability Assessment in Dementia Scale (DADS) the carer assesses the patient's ability to initiate, plan, organize and perform activities of daily living. The Rapid Disability Rating Scale is a similar 18-item questionnaire completed by the carer that combines assessment of daily living skills with measurement of ability to communicate, degree of confusion, depression and co-operativeness.

Making sense of scales and ratings

The primary reason for all these scales is to make dementia measurable. Only by being able to enumerate all the problems that occur in the disease can we apply reliable statistical methods to the results of treatments, and therefore have evidence of their effects or ill-effects.

Using scales to assess the severity and progression of dementia in a person not in a clinical trial is very much a secondary aim. Lon Schneider, of the University of Southern California in Los Angeles, puts the average family doctor's feelings about such scales well. He wrote:

> A clinician benefits from these tools [rating scales] in being able to better appreciate the presentation, severity, frequency and clinical course of problems. However, a clinician should not fall victim to the tyranny of scales and fail to assess patients clinically, or suspend his or her clinical judgement because of a rating scale score.

The fact is that, once we find that someone has dementia, and that what is needed is long-term care, not entry to a trial of new drug, most general practitioners like myself make our day-to-day decisions not on rating scale results, but on our assessment of the person's particular problems. They vary from case to case. The stage and severity of dementia become increasingly self-evident as time passes, and scales become academic, rather than a necessity.

5

How dementia (usually) progresses

Doctors learn very early on in their careers that it is foolish to try to predict precisely how a disease will develop. We can make a fair stab at how a common cold will work out, but for anything more complex, we often end up with egg on our faces. That's why I wonder, when I hear stories about someone, say, with cancer, who has been given so many months to live, who gave them that information. Almost certainly it was not the doctor. Because although statistics may set certain odds on survival times in different stages of diseases, they cannot be applied to individual cases. Women with a particular stage of breast cancer may be given a 50 per cent chance of surviving five years, but that means that many live much longer, and that a few only survive a few months.

It is similar with the dementias. Some forms of dementia show a steeper downhill curve than others. For example, my patients who have had multi-infarct dementia seem to have deteriorated much faster than those with Alzheimer's disease. However, that is just one doctor's experience with a small number of patients, albeit over more than 30 years. If we need to know, at least roughly, what is likely to happen to a person who has been newly diagnosed as having dementia, someone has to study thousands of such patients and follow them over many years.

Professor Barry Reisberg, of the Aging and Dementia Research Center in New York, has done precisely this. Barry and his team developed the Global Deterioration Scale for dementia (see page 37), based on the progression of dementia in the patients they have seen over more than 20 years. It is a useful guide to the usual progression of Alzheimer's disease, with the proviso that although most people with the disease go through the same stages of deterioration in the same order, some do so faster than others.

The Reisberg team defined seven stages of brain ageing, which encompass normal changes with age that merge into progressive Alzheimer's disease. Each stage is recognizable and measurable, and can take from two to seven years to run, so that the slow progress towards the final stage of immobility and complete loss of reason and understanding may take more than 20 years.

Stage 1 is normal brain function and normal living. In stage 2, people complain of moderate difficulties with cognition – reasoning and understanding complex problems. For example, Professor Reisberg chooses as a typical example of stage 2 an 80-year-old colleague in his laboratory who is still performing valuable skilled work, but who is exasperated at her lack of understanding of new problems and technology. This stage is defined as normal ageing.

Most people in stage 2 do not go on to stage 3. Of those who do pass into stage 3, the earliest difficulty is in handling complex tasks at work. They are usually tasks with which they have been familiar, so that workmates notice some deterioration in their efficiency. They may be slower, or making more mistakes than before.

Stage 3 is labelled by the New York team as the 'incipient' stage of Alzheimer's. Only about half of people in stage 3 progress to stage 4. Stage 3 commonly lasts around seven years, but it may be missed out altogether.

By stage 4, people are in early, or mild, Alzheimer's disease. They find it difficult to handle some of the more complex areas of normal daily living, such as their personal finances. This is the stage when they forget to pay the rent or other bills. They can no longer cope with organizing special meals for the family, like Christmas dinner. They need help to organize themselves, but they can still live at home, with carers and family looking in and supporting them.

According to Professor Reisberg, stage 4 usually lasts about 2 years, after which time most sufferers have slipped into stage 5. This is 'moderate' Alzheimer's disease. By now, they can't cope with simpler decisions in their daily lives. For example, they can't decide what to wear, so that they are in a quandary every morning. They can't manage to shop or find their way around without help. By this stage, although they may seem fairly normal on fleeting acquaintance, they no longer remember the schools they attended, the name of their head of state or government, or their own address.

Amazingly, some people in stage 5 can still manage to work and hide their mental loss. Professor Reisberg recalls an 82-year-old psychoanalyst in stage 5 who needed 24-hour assistance at home, but still had one patient in therapy! Jürgen Thorwald, in his book *The Dismissal* described in detail the dementia that affected Ferdinand Sauerbruch, the world-famous German surgeon during and after the Second World War. In the early part of the century Sauerbruch had pioneered first chest surgery, then brain surgery, at the Charité Hospital in Berlin.

By 1940 he was obviously dementing, but his Nazi superiors kept him in office, using him as a propaganda weapon. After all, if Sauerbruch could be seen to be supporting their regime, they could not be all bad. The decision was a disaster. Many people died in Sauerbruch's operating theatres, despite all the efforts of his colleagues to prevent him from working. He was eventually quietly dismissed by the Nazis, but was reinstated by the Soviet authorities when they took over. Propaganda could work for them, as much as for the Nazis.

They learned of their mistake when a high-ranking Soviet army officer died on Sauerbruch's table, and they, too, were forced to dismiss him. For months after that, Sauerbruch tried to operate at home, and such was his reputation that, tragically, people still queued at his door and died under his hands. This horrific ending to a great man's professional life was hushed up by the authorities. It remains a lesson for everyone to be vigilant, and maybe, also, for older professionals to learn to let go of the reins before their judgement goes.

Stage 5 lasts, again according to Professor Reisberg, around 18 months. By stage 6 they can't dress without assistance. They begin to lose their abilities to wash without help. They don't know how to adjust the hot and cold taps, so that they may scald themselves. As stage 6 progresses, they need a spouse or carer to help them at the toilet.

Stage 6 is when the family's burden begins to peak. By now the patients themselves are protected by their denial of the disease, although they may have occasional flashes of insight. One patient in stage 6 managed, in a rare lucid period, to write: 'Dear Doctor, I hope that you can help me snap out of this nightmare.' By the end of stage 6, patients become incontinent, and that is often the spur to admission to nursing home or hospital care.

Before describing stage 7, this may be the best point at which to expand on what happens in stages 3 to 6. One important area is denial of the illness. People complain of memory and reasoning problems when they are in stage 3. They are worried that they are losing their minds. However, that worry disappears as they slip into the later stages, so that by late stage 4 and certainly by stage 5 they often deny that there is anything wrong. This becomes a serious problem for the carers and family, so that by stage 6 the emotional problems are much worse for the spouse and carers than for the patients themselves.

Emotional changes vary from patient to patient. They are not universal, but among the most typical are accusations of theft against their nearest and dearest. This has been labelled the 'People are stealing things' scenario. The sequence goes something like this. Patients misplace an object or hide something valuable, then forget where they put them. Because they can't find them, they believe that their family is hiding them. This is followed by the delusion that people are coming into their home and stealing things. They become suspicious of everyone coming into the home, even when they are close relatives or a life-long partner.

The second major scenario is 'This house is not my home'. Patients may lose their ability to recognize familiar things. Because they can't recognize their surroundings, they become convinced that someone has taken them away from their home. They wander off, to find their old home: they may vaguely remember the details of a home they left many years before. When a spouse or other relative tries to stop them, they become violent, lashing out verbally and physically, and often injuring their well-meaning carers.

In a similar vein, they fail to recognize their children. One woman believed that a cabbage patch doll, which she carried everywhere with her, was her son, who in reality was a university professor. She became very aggressive when he tried to help her understand the truth, and he was naturally very upset that he could make no headway with her.

It is when these problems start to arise that behavioural scales (see page 39) can come in useful. They differ in detail, but they all have in common assessments of the seven main categories of behaviour problems that carers may have to face. These include:

- paranoid delusions
- hallucinations
- disorders of normal activity, such as pacing around aimlessly
- aggression
- disturbances of the normal day and night rhythm (turning night into day and vice versa)
- mood changes – mainly depression
- anxieties and phobias.

It matters little whether or not an actual score on a scale is made, as long as each of these categories is assessed, so as to quantify their burden on the carers and family. Once that is done, treatment can aim at relieving them. This is a very practical aim, as many behaviour problems can be reduced or minimized with proper management.

Severe behaviour problems start in late stage 4 and peak in stage 5. They can be better coped with if the family and carers know about the possibilities in advance. Some find it worthwhile to set up family support groups, so that they can identify how much help the patient needs at each stage.

By stage 4 the main questions to be addressed by families and carers are:

- Can the patient live alone?
- Can the patient still drive?
- How can the patient cope with being left alone?
- How can the patient cope with dressing and toilet?
- How can we as carers make life easier and more bearable for all of us, patient and carers alike?

Behaviour, at least as much as loss of intellect and reason, is important in giving the answers. Emotional and behaviour problems are by this stage the leading issues raised by families of patients to their doctors, and they are, along with incontinence, the main reason for admitting them to long-term nursing home and hospital care.

Stage 6 lasts around 2 to 3 years, then progresses to stage 7. In this final stage, speech begins to go. Fewer and fewer words are used, so that the patient repeats a phrase or words over and over again, or makes up nonsense words. Eventually only around half a dozen words, then a single word, is left. That one word finally disappears, so that all speech communication goes.

Loss of speech is followed by the loss of walking. For a while, sufferers can sit up: then even that is lost, so that they lie relatively inert. They lose their facial expressions, the last being the ability to smile. Finally, they cannot hold up their head, and they are rigid, curled up and motionless. In effect, the skills that the patient acquired as a baby are lost in exact reverse order to that in which they were learned, and much to the same timetable.

Most people succumb in the second or third year of stage 7, when they lose their ability to sit up, but tragically this last stage can sometimes last eight years or more. Barry Reisberg told me that more than half a million are in this stage, in American nursing homes. All patients with all illnesses in all forms of hospitals in the United States only number between 900,000 and one million.

I thought long and hard before writing this chapter, because it can only be very depressing for people caring for their loved ones with dementia. But I agree with Professor Reisberg's reasons for bringing it to their notice. He believes if carers and relatives have some idea of what lies ahead they can plan and cope better. For example, faced with a patient in early stage 5, carers can be fairly confident that he or she may be worse in a year's time, but is unlikely to be incontinent.

Given this timetable the behaviour problems can be anticipated and dealt with, and facilities for help put into place in advance. Most of all the family learns about the illness and its problems, understands that they are part of the illness, and that there are mechanisms in place in most communities to help to alleviate them. With the problems out in the open, and not swept under the carpet, much more can be done to help.

Of course, making the diagnosis of Alzheimer's disease places a heavy burden on everyone concerned. Most doctors, once the illness is suspected, will first see the responsible members of the family on their own, without the patient being present. At that meeting, what is likely to happen in the future is explained in detail. Only then is the patient seen. What is usually said is, 'You do have a memory problem. We are doing all we can, and may be able to offer you medicine that can help some of your symptoms.'

My own feeling is that this is kinder than telling someone that he or she has an incurable progressive disease. For most patients this seems enough, yet some demand the right to know if they have Alzheimer's or not. Once they have been given this diagnosis, it is impossible to retract what has been said, and they often regret this afterwards.

I asked Professor Reisberg at a recent meeting if the time course of the disease differs according to the age at which it started. He felt that, generally, it did not. Uncommon inherited forms of Alzheimer's disease that start earlier in life may progress more rapidly, as do forms of dementia in which there are also multiple small strokes. However, saying that the disease will run a course of around 20 years has a different meaning when talking to a 50-year-old than to an 80-year-old.

Professor Reisberg also stressed that it is only when the fourth stage is reached that one can be sure that the disease will progress. Most people never progress further than stage 3. This is why stage 3 is listed as 'incipient' Alzheimer's disease.

The Reisberg stages can be correlated roughly with MMSE scores (see Chapter 4). MMSEs in stage 2 are 29 or 30. In stage 3 the MMSE ranges from 25 to 29. By stage 4 it is around 19; by stage 5, it has dropped to 14; and at the transition from stage 5 to stage 6 it is 5. By the end of stage 6 the MMSE is 0. On the New York figures, it takes an average of seven years to travel through stage 3, and two more years to pass through stage 4. Stage 5 lasts around 18 months, and stage 6 two and a half years. Stage 7 lasts from two to eight years.

Of course, these figures are averages, so that they vary quite widely, but they do come from a very large number of people followed for many years by researchers in a highly scientific specialist department. That makes them of some use in predicting future progression in dementia and in behaviour problems.

Probably the most important reason for staging dementias in this way, however, is that their treatment varies according to the stage. People in stage 3 and early stage 4 (usually looked on as mild dementia) are candidates for drugs that may slow down the progress of the dementia. Patients in late stage 4 and stage 5 may well need treatments to deal with their emotional and behaviour problems. For people in stage 6, the main aim is to maximize good nursing, nutritional and social care. Drugs for dementia or behaviour or even mood are no longer appropriate. Those in stage 7 need 24-hour nursing care.

How these stages of treatment of dementia are managed is described from Chapter 6 onwards, and the next chapter is probably the appropriate place to describe the different types of dementia in more detail. Not all cases of dementia are of the Alzheimer's type. Although the practical problems they pose are similar to those in Alzheimer's, and their treatments are broadly the same, they do differ in some of their symptoms and in their rates of progression. Knowing how they do so, and the kind of dementia that people have, can help carers and family, and often the people themselves, to plan ahead.

6
Managing the early stages

Treating dementia depends very much on the stage the patient has reached. In the early stages the aim is to keep the patient at work and socially active as long as possible, to keep the brain as active as possible, and to try to slow down the process with modern drugs. This chapter concentrates on how to manage these early stages.

Understandably, we all fear being told we have dementia, whatever the type. It is at least as bad as being told we have cancer – probably worse, because today many people can survive cancer. Families often want to keep the news from the patient, but the doctor must, ethically (because the patient has a right to know), try to raise the subject in as tactful as possible a way. One approach is for the doctor to say, 'You have a memory problem that is caused by an illness. Would you like to know more about it?'

People who say 'no' to this, or who quickly change the subject, probably don't want to be told. They surely have a right to know their diagnosis, but they also have a right not to have it forced upon them. I have found that families are often more afraid of patients being told than the patients are themselves. Many patients are relieved that there is an explanation for their frustration and anger.

In fact, many people with early dementia know, perhaps subconsciously, that they are ill. Some deny the possibility that they are demeting, others rage and become even more frustrated after the diagnosis. This is the time for open discussion with them about how to prepare for the future. There may not be a chance later.

Once the initial reaction has settled, people with newly diagnosed dementia often appreciate the opportunity to discuss their impending difficulties. They fear not only for themselves but the burden they will put upon their families, and they start the long process of grief for what they have lost and their loss of a long-term future. They also must co-operate in the planning for the future.

The first step is for carers and patient alike to understand what is going on. They should read all they can about the illness and be helped by professionals and the societies set up for them. The most important of these is the Alzheimer's Society (ADS), which is dedicated to help people with dementia and their families, world-wide.

This is discussed later. Each country has its own ADS branch and every general practitioner knows where it is. There is usually, too, a local Alzheimer's Disease Association or Group that can be of immense practical help and works alongside the ADS.

Step two is to deal with the initial reaction to breaking the news. Families must deal with it, whether it is grief and depression, anger and frustration, or denial that the dementia exists. This last reaction can lead to 'doctor shopping', where the affected person is touted around specialist after specialist, in the vain hope that one can be found to give a different diagnosis and hold out a chance of a cure. It is hard, but please try to accept the diagnosis, and don't shop around. It is a waste of time – yours, the doctors' and the patient's.

People often react, naturally, to the news that they have dementia by going to pieces, and being completely demoralized. One way to cope with this is to make a 'Pleasant Event Schedule'. The family mulls over the activities and hobbies that the person used to enjoy, and lists them in increasing order of difficulty. (One early sign of dementia is to lose interest in a previously absorbing activity.) Then they re-introduce the one they think both the easiest and that the patient would enjoy most. Once the person finds this pleasurable, then the next order of difficulty can be faced. An example for a man might be to keep him company watching a football match on the television. The next step may be to go to the local ground to watch his favourite team. The third may even be to travel to an away game, or to watch a grandson playing for his school.

For a woman, the increasing 'hierarchy' of activities may start with tea with old friends in the house, then follow with a shopping expedition, then an afternoon out to a stately home or the seaside.

On these pleasurable activities people with dementia must always be accompanied by someone who is close and sympathetic and very familiar, who understands and reacts sensibly to any problems. The aim is to re-introduce them as far as possible to the pleasures of life that they enjoyed before their illness started. Dr L. Teri and colleagues described this approach in the *Journal of Gerontology*. This is an academic report intended for interested doctors, but it is readable by family doctors and carers. The method does seem to lift the depression that often follows the diagnosis, and this makes the underlying dementia much easier to manage.

The next subject to be faced is chances of inheriting the disease. The patients' closest relatives all wish to know their own risk of developing it. That is not yet possible. We do not have enough knowledge yet about the genetic flaws in Alzheimer's to give an accurate estimate of risk. All that we can say is that if there were several cases in previous generations, then the risk to current generations is higher if those cases started at younger ages.

Children, or brothers and sisters of people newly diagnosed with Alzheimer's disease may be reassured by looking at their chances in the following way. The risk to the general population of developing Alzheimer's disease before the age of 75 is under 3 per cent. People with parents, brothers or sisters who developed the disease after their seventy-fifth birthday have double this risk of eventually developing the disease, raising it to 6 per cent. If you have had two or more close relatives who started to have the disease before they were 65, then the risk is 12 per cent. In a very few families, in whom there are many cases spread through several generations, starting early in life, the risk to close relatives can climb as high as 50 per cent, but this is probably around two in a hundred cases in all.

Usually the next step for the doctor in charge is to call a family meeting, attended by all the day-to-day carers and the patient. At this meeting the practical consequences of the diagnosis must be discussed. This is not just about medical care and keeping the patient happy and comfortable, but about legal, financial, work-related and travel matters, and support for the carers. It is best to deal with these details at the beginning of this long journey, and not to have to cope with them suddenly in a future emergency.

It seems harsh to introduce the subject so early in the illness, but people with dementia should provide power of attorney over their finances to a person whom they trust fairly soon after the diagnosis. This is usually a spouse or a son or daughter. As the dementia worsens, they will no longer be able to understand how to manage their money, and it may not be long before they can no longer sign their name. If by that time there is no power of attorney, it can be very difficult for the family to take quick control of the finances. A guardian or financial manager may need to be appointed.

It is common for couples in the early years of their marriage to make 'mirror wills' – one spouse leaving his or her estate to the other and vice versa. That can be a bad idea. If the non-demented spouse dies first (sadly not an unknown happening), it can leave the ill partner with the impossible task of managing the estate. So while you can, make a new will, appointing someone else as executor.

51

It is also vital to recognize that, if you are caring for someone with early dementia, you may have many years to do so. So you must organize your future income to make it the maximum. That means looking for the maximum benefit on early retirement on medical grounds, sickness benefits, disability insurance payments and pension. You must seek early advice on all these things. In some countries, spouses and offspring who have to leave work to care for a sick partner or parent may get state financial help to do so.

It is wise, also, to look ahead at a possible future nursing home or sheltered housing place. Obviously, people want to stay in their own homes for as long as possible. The downside to that is that the longer the dementia continues, the more difficult it is to adjust to a new environment. People who make the move earlier adjust better to their later increased dependence on others, and good sheltered housing, retirement villages and nursing homes provide that gradual increase in care almost seamlessly. Wait too long before considering the move out of the family home, and the patient is much more likely to respond with agitation, confusion, aggression, and misery. Patient and carers together must decide when the transition from home to a cared-for environment is to take place, and take the advice of the professionals when they are making their decisions.

Two big issues also facing the person with early dementia are work and driving. Most of the routine jobs that people could continue in the past have disappeared, swept away by mechanization and our computerized society. Few people can continue with full-time employment, and still do justice to their jobs, after their dementia has been diagnosed.

However, it can be difficult to persuade people of that fact, and it seems to be more difficult the more complex the job. Academics who have 'lost the place' can be very difficult to remove. It is sometimes worse for people in jobs that directly affect the lives of others. Ferdinand Sauerbruch was by no means the only doctor with no insight into his dementia. The same goes for people who drive for a living – whether it is cars or trains. It is hard to think of professional pilots getting away with dementia in their six-monthly physical and mental tests, but doctors and salesmen and lorry drivers are not so well or so frequently regulated. It is therefore up to family and friends and anyone 'in the know' about the diagnosis to make sure that the person is absolutely of no risk to anyone, including himself or herself, by staying in the job.

Which leads us on to driving. People with early dementia hate most of all their ability to drive being taken away. They get very angry about it, seeing it as the first attack on their independence. They do not accept that they cannot continue to drive on their usual routes. The argument they often put forward, that is often even supported by their family, is that 'it would be a shame to deprive them of their last bit of liberty'.

It is true that most people with early dementia can negotiate the familiar roads around their home with little risk of accident. But that risk is still higher than with a driver with normal brain function. People with Alzheimer's disease who continue to drive, even in the earliest stages, do cause more than their fair share of accidents. This is because the disease does not just affect cognition alone. It also affects perception of place and position, slows timing and reflexes, worsens co-ordination, and limits the abilities to plan ahead and solve problems. All of these difficulties are incompatible with safe driving.

In many countries now, including the United Kingdom, it is against the law not to report someone who is driving, but is clearly unfit to do so, to the authorities. In fact, in the United Kingdom it is legally binding on people who find that they have a disease that might impair their driving to report themselves to the authorities. If there is doubt about such abilities, then a driving test will be arranged. However, because of the risk to others, dementia should be an absolute bar to driving, from the first day of diagnosis onwards.

The early stage of Alzheimer's is also the time to get in touch with your local support groups. Thanks largely to the work of the Alzheimer's Society all over the world in publicizing the need for care, and to national societies like Alzheimer Scotland and the Alzheimer Society of Ireland in providing the care, everyone has a local Alzheimer association nearby, with willing and expert helpers. Apart from providing direct support to families caring for someone with dementia, they produce newsletters, booklets and videos on practical aspects of Alzheimer's care. They counsel families and train carers, run telephone help lines and organize meetings. Many run respite services for carers in the home, day care centres and some manage nursing homes.

If you are a carer, do take advantage of the training offered by your local association. It can ease your mental stress, improve your ability to cope, your practical skills, and your knowledge of the illness, and in doing so, improve your own and your patient's quality of life. In the long run, the well-trained carer can keep their patient at home for longer and may even prolong the time spent in the earlier, less distressing stages of the disease. And when the time comes for changes to be made, they can be planned ahead and carried through with less distress.

Finally, there are prescription drugs. In theory, the new drugs designed to slow down the mental deterioration in dementia are only useful in these early stages: by the middle stages they offer no advantages. Because of this, they are reviewed in the next chapter, before we move on to the management of the later years.

7

Drug treatments for early dementia

The history of medical treatments for dementia is littered with reports of drugs that somehow, often by accident, were found to ease the symptoms or prevent its onset. The problem is that when they were subjected to well-controlled drug trials, most were found wanting.

The first medical treatments that reached public attention were anti-oxidants such as vitamin E and beta-carotene. 'Free oxygen radicals', highly active molecules produced by chemical reactions within stressed cells, have attracted huge interest in the last ten years or so, because they have been linked to damage to brain tissues in dementia, and to blood vessels in heart disease and stroke. Anti-oxidants such as vitamin E and beta-carotene were in theory good for us, because by 'mopping up' the free radicals in the tissues, such damage might be prevented.

This was great in theory, but did not turn out to be effective in practice. Several studies comparing people of similar age with and without Alzheimer's disease found that the two groups contained similar proportions of people who had taken the anti-oxidants over many years. There is therefore no hard evidence that taking extra vitamin E or beta-carotene protects against the disease.

There may be better evidence for taking aspirin, at least to prevent Alzheimer's, if not to treat it. Two large studies of people who had taken, over many years, aspirin or other anti-inflammatory drugs (such as ibuprofen, naprosyn or indomethacin) for arthritis, found that fewer of them than expected developed dementia. In a third study, previous long-term treatment with aspirin and/or anti-inflammatory drugs, but not paracetamol, also protected significantly against the onset of Alzheimer's disease. Paracetamol's lack of effect is not surprising, because it is a painkiller, and has no anti-inflammatory action. The apparent action of anti-inflammatory drugs depends on inflammation in the brain being an underlying cause of the dementia. However, the story of anti-inflammatories is not all positive. Another long-term study of anti-inflammatories failed to find an effect, good or bad, on dementia.

With these contradicting results, the effects of aspirin and its fellow anti-inflammatory drugs are still in doubt. They should be resolved by current forward-looking studies, in which whole communities have been enrolled. People without dementia have been randomly allocated to aspirin or to placebo, and are taking them for a lifetime or until they develop dementia. If aspirin significantly protects against dementia, it will be linked with far fewer cases. The Caerphilly project in Wales, for which Professor Peter Elwood of the University of Cardiff made a preliminary report in 2003, suggests that aspirin does protect against the onset of dementia, though we still need more complete results and corroboration by other studies.

Probably the best evidence for prevention of dementia, and perhaps for treating it in the early stages, comes from studies of hormone replacement therapy (HRT) for women in and after the menopause. In the United States, V. W. Henderson reported that there were fewer cases of dementia among older women using HRT than among non-HRT using women of the same age. This was followed by a report that HRT improves mood in older women and may even improve cognition.

These reports led to several theories on why HRT should be so beneficial. Evidence was put forward that oestrogen, the main hormone in HRT, promotes the growth of the cholinergic nerves in the brain, thought to be responsible for organizing memory and cognition. It also stimulates the breakdown of amyloid (see Chapter 2) and acts favourably upon apolipoprotein E, a fat-protein compound linked genetically to Alzheimer's, according to Dr Ming-Xin Tang of Columbia University, New York, and his associates. It improves the brain's efficiency in using glucose, improves the brain's circulation, and is an anti-oxidant. A formidable range of anti-dementia actions for one hormone!

The Tang team comprised experts from Columbia University, the New York State Psychiatric Institute, and two highly respected Alzheimer's Research Centres, the Gertrude H. Sergievsky Centre and the Taub Centre. They followed 1,124 elderly women initially free of Alzheimer's disease or Parkinson's disease or stroke, to detect the first signs of Alzheimer's and other forms of dementia. The age at diagnosis of dementia was much later among the 156 women who had taken HRT after the menopause, and their overall risk of developing dementia was a staggering one-third of those who had not taken it. The actual figures are astonishing: only 9 of the 156 women who had had HRT developed dementia, in contrast to 158 of the 968 women who had not had HRT. The odds for this being a chance finding are 100 to 1 against!

The timing of the HRT mattered, too. The higher the dose and the longer the women had taken it, the greater the protection. Women who had taken it for more than one year had less risk than those taking it for a shorter time. None of the 23 women who were using HRT at the time they entered the study developed dementia.

HRT's protective effect was confirmed in the well-publicized US study of tacrine (see later in this chapter), although most press reports tended to stress the effect of the new drug, rather than the HRT aspect of it. This trial showed that people with dementia taking both tacrine and oestrogen improved significantly more than those taking tacrine alone, according to Dr Lon S. Schneider of the University of Southern California. Women on either the combined treatment or tacrine alone fared much better than women given only placebo.

Despite this excellent evidence that HRT protects against dementia and may help women with early dementia, the jury is still out on how much difference it really makes to them. This must wait for the results of larger trials being conducted in several countries. However, whenever I have told my older women patients who have particular reason to fear dementia about these results they have all opted to start HRT. And I support their decision.

The American Psychiatric Association agrees with me. They include a discussion of HRT in their latest 'Practice guidelines for the treatment of patients with Alzheimer's disease and other dementias of late life', published in the *American Journal of Psychiatry*.

Obviously HRT with oestrogens is not an option for men. Men who feel left out by this, however, can take some comfort by another finding of the Tang team. Males produce small amounts of the hormone oestrone throughout their lives – there may be an emotional male menopause, but there is no hormonal one. And the male brain converts oestrone to oestrogen, so that it is virtually exposed continually to a form of local, though low-dose, HRT. This may be one reason for the slightly lower rate of non-inherited Alzheimer's disease in men than in women.

Cholinergic agents (or cholinesterase inhibitors)

The big news in drugs for dementia is the development of cholinergic drugs. The principle behind them is the finding that acetylcholine is the brain transmitter most obviously involved in the organization of memory and intellect. The more acetylcholine there is washing around the brain cells, so goes the theory, the better the memory and the sharper the cognition, or intellectual ability.

Cholinergic drugs can either stimulate the production of acetylcholine or block its breakdown: the result should be the same. However, trials of different types of cholinergic drugs suggest that this is not so. Drugs that increase brain levels of acetylcholine by reducing its breakdown seem to work better than those that increase its production. Why this is so is not clear, except that it may be more difficult to stimulate new acetylcholine production in brain cells that are already failing than to block acetylcholine destruction once the cells have produced it.

The big difference came with tacrine. Superficially, the claims that it works in dementia look modest. In a 30-week trial, compared to placebo, tacrine maintained the patients' status quo or produced mild improvement. They were about six months better off on the graph of decline in memory and cognition, according to Professor Martin Knapp of the London School of Economics and Political Science (LSE). The best effects were in patients who could tolerate the highest doses of 120mg or 160mg per day, but in fact only half of the subjects managed to finish the trial, and there were more dropouts on the higher doses. Most found that the drug upset their stomachs, and some were withdrawn from the trial because there were signs that it disturbed their liver chemistry.

Reports of tacrine use over longer periods are less reliable scientifically. They are mainly based on anecdote or observation, rather than studies in which people were allocated randomly and blindly (to doctors and patients) to different treatments. This raises doubts about possible bias, but there does seem to be some merit in its use. Among the conclusions reached by various studies are:

- in patients who respond to tacrine, the average benefit lasts for 91 weeks;
- giving tacrine at a dose of 120mg per day or more delays the time to nursing home admission for longer than a lower dose;
- people who stop taking tacrine relapse and decline faster;
- tacrine leads to less apathy, fewer hallucinations, fewer abnormal movements and reduces uninhibited behaviour.

Tacrine was just the first of a series of similar drugs with a similar biological action. The next was donepezil, given once a day (an advantage over three times a day dosage). It is claimed to be as effective as tacrine, but less likely to cause side-effects severe enough to cause people to stop taking it. Over two years, people taking donepezil kept above their initial performance levels for an average of 38 weeks. The rate of decline in intellect has been reported as slowed by the drug.

Three more cholinergic drugs, rivastigmine, galantamine and sustained-release physostigmine, have since joined tacrine and donepezil on the medical prescription lists across the world. Their results are similar. I here have to admit to close connections to another cholinergic drug, metrifonate. It showed even more promise than its rivals in its early studies, and I was asked to report on the European clinical trial results leading up to its release. Sadly, it fell at the last hurdle because of a problem trial result in the United States. I hope that this was just a 'blip' in its development and that all the research into it was not wasted.

If this news about cholinergic agents (technically, they are all properly classified as 'cholinesterase inhibitors') sounds encouraging, then it is best to temper enthusiasm with caution. They all share a battery of adverse effects, such as nausea, vomiting, coughing and tiredness, that are the direct result of raising acetylcholine levels elsewhere than in the brain. However, if the patient can tolerate them for a week or so, they usually decrease. People on long-term cholinergics, especially tacrine, should be regularly monitored for early signs of liver problems.

The American Psychiatric Association reviewed the evidence for cholinesterase inhibitors in 1997. It concluded that although the evidence suggested only a modest improvement in some patients, the absence of alternative treatment must mean that people with mild or moderate Alzheimer's disease should be offered a trial of them, provided there is no medical reason for withholding them. However, patients and their families must be advised that their potential benefits are limited, they are costly, and they can cause many and severe side-effects.

Some idea of their effect is given by a comparison between donepezil and tacrine, taken for one to two years, using as 'controls' a previous group of Alzheimer's patients followed, untreated, over a similar period. Over the 12 to 24 months of the trial, the donepezil-treated group deteriorated by around 1.5 MMSE points (see Chapter 4 for the MMSE scale). The tacrine group did not differ from the control, untreated group, who had deteriorated over the same time by around 3.3 MMSE points.

An improvement in deterioration rate measuring 1.8 MMSE points over one to two years is not much. It is still a deterioration, not an improvement, in the patient, and the slowing of the disease process almost certainly would not be seen by the family and carers. Yet over many years it may make a difference, so that people stay longer in a condition that allows them to stay at home, or at least maintain adequate independence in a sheltered environment. It may make the difference between being able to wash and use the toilet efficiently or not, at least for several months longer than would otherwise be the case. And in each clinical trial population treated with cholinergics, a few patients seem to do spectacularly well. It is only by trying the drugs that these patients will be found.

On the whole, therefore, it is worthwhile to try cholinergic drugs in people with early and moderate dementia. If they make no real difference, they can be stopped. They are unlikely to do harm. However, they will never reverse or cure dementia, and their effects are bound to fail in the end, because they depend on the brain cells' diminishing ability to produce acetylcholine. They work by stopping the breakdown of whatever amount of acetylcholine the surviving cells can produce, thereby increasing the amount of acetylcholine in the spaces around the cells. It is the between-the-cells acetylcholine that is the basis of transmission of messages from cell to cell, and that is the basis of memory and cognition. Once cells no longer produce acetylcholine, cholinesterase inhibitors have no acetylcholine to protect from breakdown, and they are no further use. So it is pointless continuing them into the later stages of the disease.

Other new drugs for dementia

Naturally, many drugs that act on the various chemical 'transmitters' in the brain (acetylcholine is just one of many such transmitters) have been tested in dementia. None have yet produced enough evidence of effectiveness to grant them a licence for use in dementia. They are mentioned here more to show the efforts being made to find something that will reverse the disease, than to promote their use in dementia. Trials of drugs that have failed are also discussed here, because people faced with the news that they, or a close relative, have dementia, often go from one suggested drug treatment to another, time after time, searching for a cure. The next pages show how futile this search can be. It is good, but sobering, to know the negative, as well as the positive.

One drug of real interest is selegiline, or L-deprenyl. This does have a licence, but for Parkinson's disease, not dementia. It belongs to the class of drugs called monoamine oxidase B inhibitors, but it may also be an anti-oxidant. Its interest lies in six well-controlled trials, five of which suggested that it produced some improvement right across the many symptoms and signs of dementia, according to Dr Mary Sano of Columbia University. In particular, it seems to make patients more active. This may be a boon or a bad thing, as it can take people out of an uninterested or relatively immobile state, so making it easier to help them, or it can just make them more anxious and agitated.

Doctors are warned to prescribe selegiline with care, especially in conjunction with other drugs, such as antidepressants and the sedative pethidine, in which it has the potential for dangerous adverse effects. So it is not a treatment to be started lightly in someone with dementia, who may already be more than usually susceptible to brain malfunction.

We already have drugs that stimulate other brain transmitters: they are regularly used in depression. The transmitters studied go by the names of serotonin, GABA, and glutamine. Sadly, drugs acting on these systems have been tried and found ineffective in dementia.

Among other approaches to dementia that have been tried and failed are the hormones somatostatin and adrenocorticotrophic hormone (ACTH), nerve growth factor (NGF), and 'nootropics'. Somatostatin and ACTH were supposed to help the brain cells to become more efficient in their processing of proteins (a fault in which might cause dementia). They did not appear to do so. Nerve growth factor is a natural substance that the body uses to prevent nerve cell death. A drug thought to stimulate NGF, sabeluzole, was no better than placebo. Nootropics are defined as drugs that protect the cells in the brain from lack of oxygen, electroconvulsant treatment (ECT), and poisoning. Three of them, piracetam, pramiracetam and oxiracetam have failed to show any effect in dementia.

Co-dergocrine mesylate (Hydergine), a drug that has been used widely for many years for dementia with no real evidence for its efficacy, is a derivative of the cereal fungus ergot. After more than a hundred studies in the elderly, it is not recommended by any national authority for dementia.

Drugs with more promise include gangliosides. Gangliosides occur in the surface membranes of normal brain cells, and are thought to protect them from damage. Because they are deficient in the Alzheimer brain, they are being given in clinical trials: we are awaiting the results. Similar trials are under way of phosphatidylserine, a normal component of brain cells that is also lacking in Alzheimer's. It may take some years yet before we know whether or not they work.

Vitamin E (also known as alpha-tocopherol) may not prevent dementia (see earlier in this chapter) but it could play a role in its treatment. The best evidence for it is a well-controlled trial in which 341 people with moderate dementia were randomly allocated to four treatment groups. One group studied by Dr Mary Sano was given placebo, one 1,000 International Units of vitamin E twice daily, one selegiline 5mg twice daily, and one received both active treatments (Sano *et al.*, 1997).

The results were quite definite, if surprising. Each of the two drugs on its own delayed the times to death, to the need to put the patient into an institution, and to a significant decline by many days (an average of 230 days for vitamin E and 215 for selegiline) compared to the placebo. But when the two were given together, the delay was much less (only 145 days). It was much more effective to give the treatments singly than to combine them. Why this should be is a puzzle, and is still being argued about. Another puzzle about these results is that none of the treatments improved the patients' performances in cognitive tests.

Because it is thought of as a vitamin, people often look upon Vitamin E as harmless. Not so. In the doses used in the trial (2,000 IU per day) it is truly a drug, not a vitamin, and can alter blood clotting mechanisms in people with bleeding problems. It must not be given along with warfarin, a drug often used in older people who have had heart surgery or thromboses (blood clots).

The American Psychiatry Association's guidelines recommend that vitamin E may be given in dementia along with a cholinesterase inhibitor such as tacrine, donepezil or rivastigmine.

Propentofylline is another drug with great theoretical potential in dementia. It is classified as a 'glial cell modulator'. Put simply, glial cells are the structural cells that lie between brain nerve cells, that are there to repair damage. One model of dementia suggests that glial cells are abnormally active, so that they release brain cell-injuring poisons such as free radicals, nitric oxide and other chemicals that cause cell death. In the laboratory, propentofylline returns abnormal glial cell activity to normal.

It was given to 901 patients with mild to moderate Alzheimer's disease and 359 patients with mild to moderate vascular dementia for up to 12 months. After that time the patients on propentofylline were markedly better than those on placebo. This was true of both types of dementia, and the drug was well tolerated.

Other drugs with less evidence for effect in dementia are listed below, mainly for completeness. They all need much more work on them before their usefulness can be proven and accepted.

The calcium blocker nimodipine is under study, on the basis that brain cells die because of a rise in their internal calcium levels. Nimodipine blocks this rise. Memantine is a drug that acts on the neurotransmitter glutamate in a way that is thought to improve memory. A Latvian study suggested that it improved people with severe dementia. Acetyl-L-carnitine may protect neurones: it needs further trials. Angiotensin-converting enzyme inhibitors (ACEIs) are used widely to control high blood pressure – they have been used in trials in dementia.

Of the popular non-pharmaceutical remedies, ginkgo biloba is probably the best known and most used in dementia. The evidence for it is not strong. The most scientific trial of ginkgo biloba was placebo controlled and patients were asked to take their allocated treatment for a year. It is true that those who took the ginkgo biloba declined less fast than those on placebo, but only half of them, and only 38 per cent of those given the placebo, finished the trial. Much more evidence is needed, preferably from other centres, before ginkgo biloba can be recommended. The same goes for another much-touted alternative medicine, melatonin.

A word about aluminium is appropriate here. For many years it was popular to link dementia to aluminium poisoning. It was claimed that the brains of dementia patients examined at post-mortem contained more than the usual amount of aluminium. Was the aluminium the cause, or the result, of the dementia? Either scenario was possible: metal poisoning could damage nerve cells, and diseased nerve cells might well take up excess aluminium.

Publicity about this scientific conundrum led many people to discard their aluminium saucepans and all aluminium food containers, and the aluminium industry has never quite recovered from the onslaught. Yet subsequent studies have shown that there is no real excess of aluminium in the Alzheimer's brain, and the aluminium theory of Alzheimer's and other dementias has long been discarded by the experts. Presumably they are now happily cooking again in aluminium pots and pans.

That theory did lead, however, to trials of the chelating agent (a chelator is a drug that removes a toxic metal from the body) desferrioxamine, in dementia. It had little effect, and it is now considered too toxic itself to be used routinely for dementia, particularly as the basis for its use is no longer accepted.

Finally, no discussion of drugs in dementia is complete without defining when to stop them. The decision to stop drug treatment is not as easy as it sounds. It need not be stopped just because the dementia is steadily worsening: the drug may still be slowing the decline, which could accelerate once it is withdrawn.

The care team should discuss stopping the drugs in three main circumstances:

- when there is no obvious benefit (or slowing of the decline) from the start of treatment;
- when the side-effects are worse than the benefits;
- and when a patient has improved on the treatment, but then declines faster, and the faster decline is noted on subsequent occasions. Carers should be aware that this faster decline may not be due to the loss of the drug effect, but because of another illness, such as an infection.

It must be said that most of the trials in dementia used people in the early or early middle stages, so that there is no good evidence that the drugs work in the later middle and final stages of the disease. So if one is to go by evidence-based medicine – the bible of modern medical practice – drugs should in theory be stopped, say, when people are ill enough to be admitted to nursing home care.

I'm not sure that I agree with this. The decision to stop drugs should take everything about the patient's care into account, and carers and family, as well as doctors and nurses, should all be involved in it. The people who spend most time with patients – those who live with them – can be particularly astute about the benefits or drawbacks of a drug. And the one trial in severely affected patients, the selegiline/vitamin E trial mentioned above, did show unexpected improvements in especially difficult patients with advanced dementia.

In the final analysis, there is no alternative to continuing a drug with a proven record unless it is having no obvious effect or doing actual harm.

Future drugs to combat inflammation

Finally, a look ahead towards possible new treatments. Earlier in this book (Chapter 2, Understanding Alzheimer's) I looked at exciting new evidence linking Alzheimer's disease and inflammatory reactions. The next step is of course finding treatments targeted at inflammation. Already research has begun into ways in which drugs might be used in the future to combat the inflammatory changes seen in the brain in Alzheimer's disease. Several different possible approaches are being explored. One of these is the use of statins, drugs often given to reduce high blood cholesterol levels. The news that statin treatment was linked to lowering the risk of Alzheimer's disease came from studies in which these drugs were primarily prescribed for people with heart disease related to high cholesterol levels. They showed that among the people given statins there were many fewer cases of Alzheimer's disease than were expected.

Statins

The widespread use of statin drugs, which has dramatically reduced the incidence of heart attack and stroke, has brought an unexpected bonus to those at risk of Alzheimer's disease. Since the drugs started to be used in different communities, it has been reported that people treated with them are at a lower than usual risk of developing Alzheimer's disease. On page 13, I mentioned a *BMJ* article by Drs Cassidy and Topol. Here is what they write:

Epidemiological studies with different study designs and patient populations have shown a 40–70 per cent reduction in the risk of Alzheimer's disease associated with statin use.

They go on to write:

> The magnitude and consistency of the effect observed is remarkable.

What has this to do with inflammation? On pages 12–14, I described how excessive deposits of cholesterol in blood vessels and in other tissues provoke a similar inflammatory reaction to those caused by bacteria and viruses. The body does not 'like' the excess cholesterol and tries to get rid of it. In the brain, the results of that inflammation may help to provoke the deposits of amyloid and the neurofibrillary tangles mentioned earlier in this book (see page 5), classic signs of Alzheimer's.

While we are not yet quite sure exactly how statins work on the brain, they seem to remove the 'bad' cholesterol from the blood, and by implication, remove the cholesterol-rich deposits of atheroma (the 'porridge' I mentioned) from the artery walls. They may do the same for the amyloid in Alzheimer's brains. However, that has not yet been proven. Statins may also work in Alzheimer's by improving the blood flow to the brain, by 'smoothing out' the artery walls, perhaps acting directly on the cells lining the smallest blood vessels in the brain to help blood flow through them more easily.

Other possible approaches

The statin story is just the beginning. Drs Cassidy and Topol describe at least five other ways in which drugs might be used in the future to combat the inflammatory changes seen in the brain in Alzheimer's disease.

Blood pressure drugs

One possible approach is to use a type of drug already widely available for lowering high blood pressure. Called angiotensin converting enzyme (ACE) blockers or angiotensin 2 blockers (A2 blockers), drugs in this group have been shown in animals to improve acetylcholine levels in the brain and to stop the accumulation of amyloid, again by damping down evidence of inflammation.

Decreasing platelet activity

Cassidy and Topol also mention that people with Alzheimer's disease could have abnormal platelets, the tiniest of the solid particles in the bloodstream intimately concerned with clotting. The platelets might have changed in a way that encourages the formation of amyloid. Making them inactive may help to slow down the process. The simplest way to do so is to use low doses of aspirin regularly or an aspirin-like drug that has a similar effect. This measure is already very successfully used for people who have heart problems or who have signs of impending stroke.

Increasing liver X receptor activity
A possible treatment that is likely to take more time to develop arises from the discovery of the liver X receptor. This structure is found on the surface of liver cells (and has also recently been found in brain cells). It controls the way the cells react to inflammatory substances such as cholesterol. The more active the receptor, the less likely the tissues are to produce amyloid, and possession of an active liver X receptor protects mice against age-related degenerative changes. A drug that activates this receptor should therefore be useful for arresting or preventing Alzheimer's disease. As Drs Cassidy and Topol write, it 'merits further study'.

Decreasing RAGE activity
RAGE stands for Receptor for Advanced Glycation End-products. In animals with diabetes, RAGEs are excessively active in response to the damage done to tissues by exposure to increased sugar (glucose) levels. Diabetes is linked to inflammation in the blood vessels and tissues, which is why uncontrolled diabetes leads to a high risk of heart attacks, strokes, kidney failure, blindness and severe reduction in the circulation of blood in the feet and legs. And, in all sorts of complex ways, RAGEs are linked to accelerated atheroma.

The association between RAGEs and diabetes in humans has been known for some years, but there is now a well-established link between RAGEs and Alzheimer's disease. Brains taken from people with Alzheimer's show three times as much RAGE activity than those from people without it. It would seem that chronic inflammation in the brain stimulates the RAGEs into extra activity, which may lead to the nerve cell damage seen in the disease. Drugs to damp down the RAGE activity in the brain are currently being studied.

Preventing angiogenesis
Finally, there is angiogenesis. This process is the development of extra blood vessels in tissue as part of the inflammatory reaction. The change is a normal part of the healing process, but it may not be

helpful in the brain, where new vessels replace nerve cells. In fact, studies of such new vessels suggest that they actively secrete a substance called peptide neurotoxic factor, which directly destroys nerve cells. Researchers have identified substances that will stop angiogenesis in cancer (similar substances are secreted by cancer cells), and this technology will certainly be considered as another possible way of arresting Alzheimer's disease.

Responding to new treatments

The really exciting news is that trials are under way on new treatments. For statins, the confirmation of any benefit they may produce concerning Alzheimer's is bound to be very slow in arriving. Controlled trials (those comparing the drugs with placebo or current treatments) would have to involve many thousands of people in the earliest stages of the disease and the drugs would have to be given for many years. Some studies have shown a 40 to 70 per cent reduction in the risk of Alzheimer's developing in individuals who were given statins. However, these results are from people given the drugs for other reasons (to prevent heart disease or stroke, for example), and who had no Alzheimer's when they started the treatment. That is, the people who were put on the statins were 40 to 70 per cent less likely to develop Alzheimer's than those who had been given the placebo (dummy) drugs. Although this evidence is not complete proof that statins actually produce this benefit, the numbers involved are so large that the results must be taken very seriously. Doctors are currently considering giving statins to people aged 50 and over who are at high risk of developing Alzheimer's disease. However, they have not yet started routinely giving the drugs for this purpose.

If inflammation is a cause of Alzheimer's, then one simple way to treat it may be with anti-inflammatory drugs. The main candidates in this group of drugs are aspirin and non-steroidal anti-inflammatory drugs (NSAIDs), such as indomethacin, ibuprofen and naproxen. The results from controlled trials have been mixed, as with those from statin trials, probably because the people studied were in the late stages of the disease and the drugs were not used for enough time. Aspirin certainly works in preventing coronary heart disease and strokes, and even in low doses it may have an anti-inflammatory action in the brain. NSAIDs may be even more efficient in doing this, but their effectiveness has yet to be proven. A similar group of drugs, the coxibs, could also be useful for preventing brain inflammation.

But the real breakthroughs may come with newer drugs that have potentially more powerful anti-inflammatory action in the brain. Many of them are already in use for heart disease and high blood pressure. More are being developed. I have mentioned ACE inhibitors and A2 blockers. Others include PPARg agonists (peroxisomal proliferator activating receptor stimulators), ACAT inhibitors (acyl Co-A cholesterol acyl transferase blockers) and thienopyridines. I believe that in the next few years we will hear a lot more about these drugs.

All the energy currently being devoted to unravelling the complexities of Alzheimer's disease is very encouraging, and I hope that this new information will give you, too, a strong sense of hope.

8
Managing the middle stages of dementia

Frankly, the middle stages of dementia are almost always the worst for carers and family. This is the time of real change in their patient. People entering middle stage dementia begin to lose insight into their condition, so that a state of relatively benign co-operation becomes one of confusion, often aggression and suspicion, and then deterioration in the ability to care for themselves, even in what seems to be the simplest actions.

These are now two patients for the doctor to look after: the person with dementia and the closest carer, who has to bear the burden of the new circumstances. This requires huge support from the whole dementia team for both of them. Patients in this stage still need to be able to talk to anyone who will listen and give sensible advice on how to cope with all the small things that seem constantly to be going wrong. Details of who can help and how are explained in Chapter 15. As the illness progresses, they are less able to follow the advice, but the caring team still needs the patience to keep on trying.

This is where the local Alzheimer's Association, and the local community services, provided in the United Kingdom jointly by the Departments of Health and of Social Services can really 'kick in' with help. For my part I must recommend our area, in Dumfries and Galloway, where the two services have moved into the same building and cut all red tape between them, so as to build a problem-free system to care for people with dementia and brain injuries. I'm happy to add that many other areas in Britain are now following their lead.

As the person becomes more and more dependent, these services can help the family to deal with finances, mobility, transport to care centres, cooking and meals, housework and other home mainten-ance. They can provide sitters-in to let the carer out, not just for shopping, but visits to friends and for other entertainment. It is not disloyal to enjoy an evening by oneself or with friends at the cinema or theatre, or a day away in the country.

Carers need time off more than ever in this stage, because the personality changes can be horrendous. They take the form of two main types of change – an over-emphasis or a loss of the person's previous characteristics. Henry Brodaty, Professor of Psychogeriatrics of the University of New South Wales in Sydney, describes these changes as caricaturing or flattening of the personality.

Caricaturing, Professor Brodaty proposes, is the result of changes in the frontal part of the brain, and can cause sexual over-activity, impulsive behaviour, coarseness and a general loss of the normal social inhibitions. Flattening, he says, is a gradual erosion of the personality, so that the person's individual characteristics, that made him or her a loveable spouse and parent, are gradually lost, and apathy takes over. The two types of personality change, opposite as they seem, can actually overlap.

It is not surprising, and completely understandable, that carers and close family become very distressed by these changes. In Professor Brodaty's words, 'they have lost the person they loved, and acquired a stranger that they do not like much'. These feelings can be eased if they are known about beforehand, but they are sometimes impossible to cope with completely. This is a time of maximum need for psychological, as well as practical, support.

It is also the time that behaviour problems arise. Having lost insight into their illness, people with middle stage dementia become very demanding, often to the point of exhausting their carers. They constantly ask questions that are answered over and over again. They alternate between abusing their carers and clinging to them, obsessively. They become aggressive physically and verbally, often resorting to shouting and screaming. They wander around the house, and outside, if they cannot be kept in. They turn night into day, wandering in the middle of the night. They lose their normal eating habits, so that they may snack between refused meals, and demand breakfast, lunch and dinner at completely the wrong times of day. And then they become incontinent.

Reading that last paragraph again, people in the process of starting to look after someone with early dementia will be convinced that they are approaching a nightmare with no respite or solutions. Yet that isn't necessarily the case. It is important first to understand that you will get help, if you ask for it. You are not alone, and you must not try to do everything on your own. That is impossible. Some doctors have described a 'martyr' syndrome among some carers, who stubbornly wish to keep strangers out of their house and want to do all the caring by themselves.

I have met a few such martyrs myself. Sometimes they respond to reason eventually, but often the person with dementia (usually a relative but often just a lifelong friend) only gets the real care that is needed once the carer falls ill, or even dies. That can be a huge trauma for the patient, in effect a double loss, of carer and of home environment at the same time. Because inevitably the patient needs immediate admission to a strange nursing home or hospital.

Family doctors have a name for this tragedy – the 'creaking gate' syndrome. In a household with a carer and a patient, the creaking gate, the patient, outlasts the gate that has never made a noise, the carer. If someone from the caring services is visiting daily, impending illness in the carer can usually be identified and dealt with in time. There is nothing worse in medical practice than having to break down a front door, knowing that there must be a disaster inside that could have been avoided by a carer being more willing to accept help.

Often this is not the carers' fault. They may be intimidated by the patient's absolute opposition to allowing anyone else in the house. Carers are often made to feel guilty at the very thought of needing a stranger to help, and to feel inadequate that they can't cope by themselves, so they carry on, wishing that they could get support, but fearing the wrath they may face if they try.

This is the time, therefore, that carers must take over the reins and all the decisions. The patients must be forced, if necessary, to accept a daily invasion into their privacy, for their carers' sakes. The silent gate must make a noise at last.

So what help is on offer? The first step is to accept advice from the local practice nurse and the Alzheimer's Association on how to cope with the new behaviour problems. That involves going over each of them in detail, trying first to understand why they arise, and then to change them, if possible. The carer can start to keep a diary of the unwanted behaviour, to chart where and when it starts, what its possible causes might be, and put forward ideas on how it can be approached. Professor Brodaty calls this the 'A, B, C' approach – Antecedents, Behaviours and Consequences.

Among the main behaviour disturbances are aggression, wandering, screaming, sleep disturbances, agitation, apathy, loss of the normal sexual inhibitions, and eating disturbances. Each is susceptible to ABC. How they can be managed is described next.

Aggression

One example Professor Brodaty gives is the finding, from such a diary, that a person becomes aggressive while being showered. In the past, a general practitioner hearing that a patient has become aggressive would reach for the prescription pad, and write down the name of a sedative. The carer then had to face a half-sleepy, but even more confused patient who became angrier still when alert enough to express the anger.

Professor Brodaty's solution is to try instead a different strategy for the time in the shower. The objection may be to the person doing the washing: it is much easier for some people not to feel embarrassed in front of a professional carer like a nurse than in front of a close relative or long-standing friend. On the other hand, some much prefer a close relative, like a spouse, to supervise their washing, and are embarrassed by an outsider. Either way, they react in the only way they know how to the circumstances – with aggression. Switching the person doing the washing, showering or bathing is therefore the first step.

Even that may not be needed. The problem may even be solved just by moving the time of the shower, perhaps from morning to evening, or switching to a bath, or to a wash down at the sink. Most of the time, simple changes like this can avoid the onset of the aggressive reaction. It is rarely possible to talk with people with dementia about why they react so aggressively to such a seemingly harmless domestic event, so trying to persuade them that they shouldn't do it is hopeless. It is often a matter of trying different solutions, haphazardly, until the right one is found.

So the aim is to try to find the triggers for the patient's outbursts of aggression, and if possible to change it or avoid it. That is greatly helped by providing the patient with surroundings that are constant and familiar, and to adjust them to suit the patient. Never try to adjust the patient to the surroundings!

Above all, says Professor Brodaty, keep communications simple, specific and slow, and show the patient by pointing to, or miming, what is needed of them. Simply telling them can instigate aggressive reactions, because by this stage many patients cannot understand verbal messages, even simple ones. Remember that they tend to think in pictures, rather than words, and that pictorial representation of tasks is much easier for them to follow than words.

Sometimes all that is needed to curb this sort of behaviour is the right type and right amount of stimulation. Deprive normal people of any age of stimulation of the senses for some time, and they will become confused. Imagine how much worse it is for people whose brains are already damaged by the dementing process.

Many nursing homes pay lip service to stimulation, by sitting people around a television set. Next time you visit one, note how many of them are asleep or are obviously oblivious of the programme. Bingo games are fine, but how many of the residents still know what the numbers are? Music is fine, too, but have the listeners got their hearing aids on?

Giving people with middle stage dementia something that interests them is often of real benefit, not just to them, but to the carers, who can join in and feel that they are doing something worthwhile. The brain does not deteriorate in all its sensory abilities equally fast: the parts of the brain receptive to music, according to Professor Brodaty, seem to be more resistant than most to decay. So music comes top of the list in stimulating value. It is best to use the music that the person preferred when he or she was well. Offering 'pop' to someone previously devoted to classical music could be a big mistake. It would enrage many normal people, never mind the person with an exaggerated emotional response.

Dancing and other physical exercise are next on the list. These keep both mind and body active, and can be indulged in by carer and patient together – always a bonus. My colleagues who take John for his golf (see Chapter 1) knew nothing of Professor Brodaty's work, but they were practising what he preached, to the letter.

People who are dementing need emotional and physical contact, too. They need to be touched, stroked, cuddled and massaged. Just because their mental skills are impaired does not diminish their emotional needs. They need to smell pleasant things, like perfumes and favourite foods. They should be presented at table with their favourite meals in an attractive way, and not served with pap just because it is easy to chew and swallow. Aromatherapy is a great new way to stimulate people: it won't in any way alter the course of the dementia, but will make it easier to bear for both carer and patient.

A pet is a great bonus, if it can be tolerated and cared for properly. I favour a cat, because it takes so little maintenance (you don't have to take it for a walk). It sits easily on a lap for hours, without feeling like a ton weight, and responds so well when stroked. When the patient makes the cat purr, it helps both animal and human alike. I also favour relaxation therapy. That can take the form of simple yoga exercises or the Alexander technique, developed in the early 1900s by an actor initially, it is said, to help his stage fright. In the simplest way, this technique teaches the person to relax and stretch every muscle, while calming the mind. The simplest Alexander exercise is to lie on one's back on the floor, head resting on a book so that the neck is straight, and stretch alternate arms and legs as far as possible, before relaxing them. If it doesn't work for the patient, it certainly will for the carer. There are Alexander teachers in most communities.

Then there is Snoezelen. Snoezelen is a word derived from Dutch words for sniffing and dozing, and was developed in the Netherlands in the 1990s. Snoezelen stimulates the senses with changing coloured lights, armchairs to relax in, vibrating cushions, perfumes and other pleasant smells, and a soap bubble machine! Most Alzheimer's Associations can organize Snoezelen for people who feel that it might help.

I would add two more techniques that often seem to help people quieten down after an episode of aggression, but that are also vital for anyone in these middle stages of dementia, aggressive or not. They are reminiscence therapy and memory training. The more content and less confused within the environment a person is, the less likely is behaviour to be bizarre. Both of these systems help the patient to find that contentment.

Reminiscence therapy uses old photographs and memorabilia from times past, like newspaper cuttings and films, to bring back memories and even for the patient to relive their early experiences. Often they are from times long before their carers existed, so it can be fascinating for carer and patient alike. Reminiscence may not have the scientific blessing of a clinical trial result to prove its efficacy, but it certainly seems to keep people happy, as long as the carers maintain an obvious interest in what they are saying. They may have heard stories about the war a million times, but listening to them again helps the patient, and that is a valid reason for doing so.

Memory training is popular across Europe. It seems to be less popular in the United Kingdom, but that may be because it wasn't invented here. Many Alzheimer's groups are now advocating it, with reasonable success. It has several features. One is to encourage the patient to concentrate on one new item at a time: this is known as 'one-tracking'. Another is to combine learning something with an action appropriate to it, like switching on the television set to the chosen station. Yet another is to use what is left of the patient's professional knowledge to bolster his everyday confidence. Specialist knowledge may be the last of the cognitive functions to go, and patients who can still remember some of their past expertise are encouraged to hold on to it for as long as possible. That may help them to hold on, too, to other reasoning powers, at least for a while. Every little advantage matters.

Memory training is aided by putting labels on absolutely everything! A diary with large print, so that every important action is listed, a large watch showing the day and date, message pads by the telephone and door, shopping lists stuck to the fridge door are all vital aids. So are room titles on doors, such as 'kitchen', 'toilet', 'bathroom', 'lounge', 'utility room', and 'bedroom', preferably with simple, glaringly obvious pictures of the usual activity inside them. This 'orienting' system prevents much confusion, and therefore, much frustration and aggression. It may seem silly and infantile to have such labels stuck all over the house, but it is very worthwhile, and neighbours and other visitors will always understand, once they know the reason.

Naomi Fell, an American expert on communicating with people with dementia, coined the phrase 'validation therapy'. She stresses that the main need is to help people with dementia keep their dignity, and to be in total sympathy with them. If they believe that they are living in a time long past, and in a different place, then they should be supported in those beliefs, rather than be brought back abruptly to today's reality. This can be used to resolve past problems and conflicts that may be their constant underlying worry. Validation therapy is used in individual, one-to-one sessions, and in groups, where it is often combined with massage or dance.

Dr Fell puts her philosophy precisely: it is 'listen to the music, not the words'. The patient's actions and emotions matter more than what is said. She is repeating, in a different way, the feelings of our Stirling poet, John Killick (see page 96). It is a message that bears repeating, again and again.

All these treatment systems are ways to ease the behaviour problems in dementia. They aim to resolve the problems that lead to aggressive behaviour in particular, but they also can help to reduce other types of behaviour pattern, such as wandering, screaming, and agitation. However, there are specific ways to deal with them, to be used alongside the above techniques.

Wandering may appear to be aimless, but it often has a very specific goal. A common one is the search for a lost spouse or child. It may be just another symptom of anxiety, or part of the picture of depression. A report from the University of Massachusetts by J. M. Swearer showed that more than half of all people with Alzheimer's are restless for much of the time, one-third pace up and down, and one quarter go wandering. So people who care for 'wanderers' are not alone. Wandering is difficult to control, so the environment has to be changed so that the wanderer comes to no harm. Music therapy and involving the wanderer in creative activities may help; there is no evidence that drugs do so.

Screaming is much commoner in institutions than in people living still at home. It drives everyone around the screamer mad. The screams may just be a frustrated person's cry for help, but at times they are caused by pain or depression. The aim is to identify the cause, if possible, and put it right. Some researchers have used behaviour-correcting systems on screamers, such as giving complete attention to them when they do not scream, and ignoring them when they do. That seems a long and difficult process. I am not sure that it either works or can be applied easily without disturbing everyone else in the room, or even the building.

Pain and depression also underlie many sleep disturbances. People with Alzheimer's disease usually get enough sleep: their problem is that it often is at the wrong time. Up to two-thirds of all people with dementia develop sleep disturbances that range from night-time restlessness to full night-and-day reversal. Attending to underlying pain, depression and other physical disease that may disturb sleep, such as bowel, bladder and stomach complaints, may help a lot. The last resort is sleeping tablets, which usually work, but compromise the already diminished ability to think normally the next day.

Many carers would like their aggressive and agitated spouses and parents to become apathetic and indifferent. They think of this behaviour as giving them a rest – until they are faced with it. Then they worry because they can no longer communicate with their partner, friend or parent, who no longer takes any initiative, shows any affection or any interest in anything. This overall lack of interest is probably a fault in the frontal part of the brain, and is quite separate from the general deterioration in memory and cognition. Little can be done to improve it, except for, perhaps, a very well organized daily routine.

Eating problems, too, are difficult to manage, presumably because they, too, indicate damage to a particular part of the brain. They vary from inability to manage knives, forks and spoons, to over-eating and to eating only the same food, day after day. Carers need patience to deal with them, and may have to adjust what they present to patients to satisfy their needs. Trying to introduce something new and interesting, that the patient might have liked in the past, may help.

A discussion on behaviour would not be complete without mentioning sex. Most people in the middle stages of dementia have given up on sex: this is probably the first area in which they become apathetic. On the other hand, a minority lose their normal sexual inhibitions, and this can become very difficult. This, too, has been linked to problems with the frontal area of the brain, and a version of it has also been reported in people whose temporal lobes (the part of the brain under the temples) are affected.

Sometimes sexual problems can be managed by applying all, or at least many, of the methods described under the paragraph on aggression. However, the last resort for men who exhibit these sexual problems are drugs to remove their sex drive. These include anti-androgen or female sex hormones.

So far, this chapter on the middle stages of dementia has not touched upon mental illness. That is perhaps strange, because in the popular use of the word, being 'demented' equates not to loss of memory or intellect, but to being 'mad' or 'insane'. No-one with any medical or nursing training would use the word in this way. However, it does highlight one problem that often arises with dementia – psychiatric illnesses. They deserve a chapter on their own, and it is appropriate that it comes next, because they appear mostly in the middle stages of dementia.

9

Psychiatric illness in dementia

The behaviour problems described in Chapter 8 are not manifestations of true psychiatric illnesses. They are direct reactions, mainly due to frustration, to the conditions in which people with dementia find themselves. They need treatments that are based more on common sense and understanding than on medical diagnosis. However, in the middle years of dementia, many people also suffer from true psychiatric illnesses, of which one is depression and the other is a syndrome that includes delusions, hallucinations and 'misidentification'. How they present and how they are managed is explained in this chapter.

Depression

It is difficult to distinguish between true depression and the dementing process, for several reasons. One is that it is difficult to find out how people with dementia feel, because they can no longer express themselves easily. They also tend to forget their symptoms, so that the normal questions that would lead a doctor to diagnose depression are not answerable. But the main difficulty is that dementia and depression share the same range of problems, such as apathy, poor memory and concentration, disturbed sleep, lack of motivation, withdrawal from contact with friends, anxiety, loss of appetite, weight and of sex urge, and the loss of pleasure in life.

So is it really important to make the second diagnosis of depression, when the first diagnosis, of dementia, is obvious? The answer must be an emphatic yes – because in many cases, treating the depression lifts the patient's mood and may also vastly improve memory and cognition. It also helps the carers, who have been reported to be much more distressed when their dementia sufferer is also depressed, according to Professor Brodaty, whose work I mentioned in the previous chapter.

Depression is suspected if the person seems more affected and low than the stage of the dementia warrants. Clues to the problems being due to depression include:

- a relatively sudden start to the change in mood and other symptoms;
- a personal history of depression before the onset of the dementia, or of close relatives with depression;
- loss of social involvement with others out of proportion to the loss of intellect or memory.

In depression, the low mood is mainly in the mornings: in dementia it tends to be the same throughout the day.

The modern treatment of depression in otherwise normal people combines drug treatment with psychological and social management. Dementia makes both these choices more difficult. For example, drugs for depression in dementia must be chosen with care. If the patient has responded to a particular drug for depression before the onset of the dementia then that can be tried again. However, the choice of a new drug usually rules out the standard 'tricyclic' antidepressant drugs, such as imipramine and doxepin, because of their side-effects.

Instead, one of the more modern antidepressants is usually tried first. They are divided into different groups, depending on the chemical systems in the brain upon which they act. None has been proved to be more effective than any other, and they do seem to help people with both depression and dementia. Among them are:

- sertraline, paroxetine, fluoxetine, citalopram and fluvoxamine
- venlafaxine, moclobemide
- tranylcypromine
- trazadone and nefazadone.

These have different doses and side-effects, so anyone looking after someone put on one of these drugs should study the product leaflet carefully, and discuss the possible problems with the doctor in charge.

Among the social therapies that have been reported as helping depression in dementia are use of the Pleasant Events Schedule and all the other social and personal support systems described in Chapter 6. Reminiscence therapy, music and dance, massage and aromatherapy, affectionate touching, compliments, and validation therapy all have their place just as much to help depression as in dementia.

Being in pleasant surroundings, eating favourite meals, being asked to take part in interesting activities, with opportunities to meet friends and, alternately, to enjoy quiet and peaceful moments, are all part of the anti-depression approach. But they are a complement, rather than an alternative, to drug therapy.

Delusions, hallucinations and misidentification

More disturbing to most carers than depression, because the symptoms are more obvious and more distressing, is the syndrome of delusions, hallucinations and misidentification. These are signs of psychosis, rather than the neurosis that is depression, and are probably why the word dementia has come into common parlance as meaning madness.

About one in three dementia patients develops them in the middle stages of the disease. The delusions mostly involve the feeling that people are stealing from them or are unfaithful. They are understandable: people with dementia may misplace valuables and think they have been stolen. They feel unattractive to their spouses, so that whenever they are separated for however short a time, they imagine that their spouses are having an affair.

Hallucinations affect about one in every four people with middle stage dementia. They usually take the form of seeing or hearing things. Misidentification syndromes, which also affect around a third of patients, take four distinct forms. They can cause patients to believe that someone close to them is an impostor, or that their own face in the mirror is not their own, but a stranger's. They misinterpret events, say, in a film or television as real, and they are convinced that the house contains a non-existent lodger.

How does one treat these phenomena? Should they be treated at all? Maybe not. If the patients themselves are not bothered by their hallucinations and delusions, there may be no point in trying to change them. If the carers can be persuaded to let them be, there may be no harm in them. It is a different matter if the patient is distressed by them.

Sometimes they are fairly easy to correct. Hallucinations and delusions can result from problems with eyesight and hearing, and can be put right by supplying a hearing aid or new glasses. Removing the mirror (they may not recognize themselves) and removing the television may avoid confusion. It is often just a noise to them. Improving patients' self-esteem by reassuring them, being affectionate towards them, and praising them may be enough to make them easier to live with.

Again, as with all problems in dementia, drugs are the last resort. 'Anti-psychotic' drugs have been developed to deal with delusions and hallucinations, but their main use is in younger people with schizophrenia. How effective they are for people with dementia is debatable. And they do have side-effects that cause particular concern for older people, who may have problems with blood pressure, for example, that are rare in younger adults.

Anti-psychotic drugs are classified as being of low or high potency. Among the low potency drugs are chlorpromazine and thioridazine. They are effective in reducing psychotic symptoms, but they add side-effects like sudden drops in blood pressure on standing ('postural hypotension'), sedation (which worsens memory and cognition) and 'anticholinergic' effects (like blurred vision, dry mouth, constipation, and in men with prostate enlargement, urinary retention).

The high potency anti-psychotic drugs, which include haloperidol, trifluoperazine and fluphenazine, produce 'extrapyramidal' side-effects, which include uncontrollable muscle jerking, tremor and difficulty in co-ordination. Newer anti-psychotics such as risperidone and olanzapine are claimed to be as effective as the older ones, but with fewer side-effects: unfortunately, comparative trials of any of these drugs in people with dementia and psychiatric problems have not been carried out.

For my part, I feel that the fewer drugs that are given in the middle stages of dementia the better. If the symptoms can be controlled by extra care and understanding, that is fine. Anti-psychotic drugs are very definitely the very last resort.

10

Coping with the later stages

There comes a time when the person with dementia must be cared for 24 hours a day, and the carers and family must face the prospect of transfer to permanent nursing home care. As mentioned previously, it is often better to do this before it becomes a matter of crisis management, and when the person with the dementia can still have some say in what is happening. However, this is not always possible, for many reasons, not least an economic one, in that long stay care is very costly, and most of the burden falls on the patient's estate.

Paradoxically, as patients enter the later stages, they become easier to look after. Their earlier behaviour and psychiatric problems recede as they become first chair-bound then bed-bound, they become less communicative, and they respond less to any form of stimulus. However, it may take all this time for the carer to come to terms with what has been happening. The grieving process may hit hard, and life-time partners may begin to fear being left alone. They need more support than ever during this final phase.

Patients by this time need to be dressed, washed, taken to the toilet, have their incontinence seen to, be fed and transferred manually around the house. They stop talking, walking or moving of their own volition, and it needs someone trained in helping them to move them from bed to chair and from armchair to toilet seat or dining chair. Local authority community services may be able to help by providing care assistants, but in most countries the dementia burden is so great that many people must rely on their own ability to pay private organizations to provide them.

The progression of dementia from this stage onwards is exactly the reverse of a child learning its skills over the first five years of life. Control of bladder and bowel is lost, followed by loss of language and mobility. Speech becomes monosyllabic, until the last word is lost. The patient can no longer walk, and becomes bedridden. Special nursing care is then needed, until the final stage in which the fetal position is assumed, and death brings much welcome relief.

If end-stage care can be organized in the home that is fine, but it entails a shift system of nurses to provide care round the clock. It is impossible for any family to manage this, without such professional help, for more than a short time. Most people who reach these final stages need the care that can only be provided in a good nursing home. The change most likely to force the patient into residential care is the onset of both urinary and faecal incontinence. Although there are excellent systems, such as adult incontinence pads and special bedding, for dealing with both types of incontinence, it is rare for even the closest of families to be able to stomach what has to be done for more than a short time.

Other developments that tend to precipitate people with dementia into residential care are failure to deal with or minimize problem behaviour (see Chapter 8), and the patient's inability to recognize the carer, with all that this means in difficult patient behaviour and distress for the carer. The other main cause of people with dementia being removed to permanent residential care is the illness or death of the carer. As mentioned earlier, this is not uncommon when the carer has been under huge and constant stress.

People who feel that they can no longer care for their parent or spouse may postpone the day because they fear criticism from the rest of the family (who usually have not contributed much directly to the care). This is very unfair, because end-stage nursing of beloved parents or spouses can replace the good memories with the nightmare ones of all the cleaning and bathing and hourly turning that are necessary. It is far better to place these burdens on the professionals in the right environment, and keep the better memories intact. Absolutely no-one, no matter how closely related, can criticize that decision. Nor should anyone ever feel guilty about making it.

The right environment should be chosen with care. Here is Professor Brodaty's list of nursing home needs:

- a home-like atmosphere and no institutional appearances and fixtures;
- décor designed to retain and stimulate memories of decades past;
- easy visibility by staff of residents from every part of the building;
- spaces for informal social gatherings and meetings;
- spaces for privacy;
- secure grounds for wandering;
- landscape designed to stimulate such as a scented garden and walks with shrubs and hedges;

- personalizing every person's living space with as much privacy as possible;
- exit doors that are disguised or difficult to open (to avoid wandering outside);
- bathroom fittings designed for various physical handicaps.

Nursing homes with all these facilities are still thin on the ground, although they are increasing in number now that they are inspected and controlled. First impressions can sometimes be misleading. Some nursing homes look so clean that they are clinical, rather than homely: this may be the sign that there is little time for personal care or for activities to stimulate the residents. Others may need decorating but be full of staff who enjoy their time with their charges. One figure that indicates a good nursing home is the staff-to-resident ratio. The higher it is, usually the more time the staff have to spend on the patients.

Families caring for people with dementia at home must plan well ahead, and that means asking questions and visiting all the potential homes in the district. The local Alzheimer's group will help with facts and opinions. Doctors and social workers will lend their views. There may be a local consumer group booklet assessing the nursing homes in your region.

Entering a nursing home should be a seamless procedure for continuing medical and nursing care. The medical and nursing notes must go with patients, and if possible, the same family doctor should continue looking after them. If that is not possible (it may be outside the doctor's area) then the new doctor must have all the information needed to continue care without delay. That means transfer of all the records and a summary of the current state of the patient and treatment for the new team.

As well as checking that this has been done, the family can help by telling the new nursing staff as much as possible, for the record, about the patient. That should include the whole life history, so that nurses can discuss the past, and understand what the patient was like before the illness. The new room should contain special mementoes, such as family photographs, favourite ornaments, perhaps the patient's own bedspread, as far as possible arranged in the way they were at home. A visitor's book to remind the patient (or the nurses) who called and when can be a talking point and a good aid to memory. The family should talk regularly to the nursing staff about how the patient is settling in and on what is needed, week by week and day by day. This keeps both family and patient feeling that the connections are being maintained, despite the watershed of removal from home.

Residential care is not always a nursing home. At the minimal care level, it is a sheltered house or a place in a retirement village. Then there are places in which the residents are still reasonably independent in self-care, but need meals and activities provided for them alongside others. The staff in such homes may supervise bathing and dressing.

Nursing homes are the next stage onwards: they look after people who need help with dressing, washing, bathing and with the toilet. People in the final stages of dementia or with untreatable behaviour problems are cared for in special dementia care units, that may be separate buildings or part of nursing home complexes. Such units specialize in managing wanderers and people who scream, without having to disturb others.

As the final days approach, the family may be faced with the choice of what should be done for the semi-conscious, immobile person who can no longer swallow. Should feeding be continued by tube, inserted through the nose, or by a gastrostomy (a tube inserted under anaesthetic by a surgeon into the stomach via the abdominal wall)? Or should the patient be allowed to die quickly, with no food, under sedation? These are decisions that cannot be taken just by the nursing or medical staff: families must face up to the fact that they have to take this responsibility squarely on their own shoulders.

Death of the person with dementia is not the end of the family doctor's involvement with the family. Most doctors, in my experience, will see the family from time to time afterwards to check that they are coping with their grief. The people who are most affected are the carers who gave up their personal life and their careers to look after the deceased, and who now find that their life is empty and their careers gone. It is a very difficult time for them. Long after the death of the dementia patient, many carers still need professional and family support. This is why Chapter 14 is devoted to caring for the carers.

11

Some famous cases

Alzheimer's disease picks out the famous and the powerful just as much as the rest of us. Riches and intellect are no protector. And sometimes they soldier on in positions of extreme power regardless of the effects they may have on the people around them. Someone with Alzheimer's in the wrong place at the wrong time can alter the course of history. Take the case of Woodrow Wilson, American President during the First World War. His brain damaged by a series of small strokes, perhaps linked to Alzheimer's disease, he was unable to make even the simplest of decisions: it is said that his wife (of course, unelected to her office as First Lady) took over all responsibility for running the country.

Woodrow Wilson clung to office – it may be said his wife clung to it for him. His namesake, British Prime Minister Harold Wilson, took a more honourable course. He resigned office just after his sixtieth birthday in 1974, when everyone accepted that he was at the height of his career. Denis Healey, Chancellor of the Exchequer at the time, wrote in his autobiography in 1990 about Harold Wilson's decision: 'He told me in the lavatory outside the Cabinet room just before informing the whole of the Cabinet on 16 March, so I was just as flabbergasted as nearly all the rest of my colleagues. His inexplicable resignation honours list gave rise to rumours that there was some personal scandal behind his resignation.'

There was no scandal. That honours list (it included favours to personal friends and dubious businessmen) may have been one indicator of the erratic judgement that is a feature of early dementia. The fact that Mr Wilson had Alzheimer's was only made public just before his death in the mid-1990s, 20 years after his resignation. Did he go because he was told that he was developing Alzheimer's? It is rumoured in medical circles that he did, and it is typical of the man that he would do so.

Just as important to late twentieth-century history is the case of Ronald Reagan. Everyone remembers, surely, the simple verbal mistakes he made when he had no autocue. The most infamous was when he welcomed Princess Diana to the United States as 'Princess David'. Around that time, his lack of intellect was being lampooned weekly in *Spitting Image* (the satirical television puppet show) in a long-running sketch in which the CIA were always looking for the President's brain. Eventually, after many episodes, it was found in a bowl of shelled walnuts – and before the surgeons could replace it in his skull, he had eaten it by mistake. All great farce and a biting comment on the times, and on the public image of the President. Sadly it was too near the mark – even during his presidency the signs of Alzheimer's disease were becoming all too apparent to those in the know. That 'Princess David' lapse was just one of many small signs that things were beginning to go wrong.

Soon after he returned to private life, after what most Americans accept as two highly successful terms of office, Ronald Reagan told America that he had Alzheimer's disease. He seemed to be a genuinely decent man, open and generous. Certainly, he and Nancy Reagan ploughed many millions of dollars into his Foundation for Research into Alzheimer's Disease. At the age of 93, after a 10-year battle with Alzheimer's, Reagan finally succumbed to pneumonia, a complication of the disease.

Whatever one thinks of his political views, President Reagan seems to have been a pleasant and gentle person all his life. Possessing this type of character before one develops the disease can be a great help to the carers, because it usually continues during the years of decline.

That was surely the case for Dame Iris Murdoch – one of the most important novelists of the twentieth century. Read *Iris*, written by her husband John Bayley, to understand how Alzheimer's can be faced by a couple, and, although the battle was eventually lost, how they triumphed over the disease. In the book, which was written when she was in the final stages of the disease, John Bayley writes about her: 'She is not sailing into the dark. The voyage is over, and, under the dark escort of Alzheimers, she has arrived somewhere. So have I.'

John and Iris met in 1954 at an Oxford College. The book describes their everyday life. Their house was too untidy for them to be able to employ a cleaning lady. They would swim in the ponds and streams they found in their country walks. They shared an all-encompassing love and mutual understanding. And that comfortable feeling of being together, despite their domestic chaos, stood them in good stead when Iris began to lose her intellect and was no longer able to write.

John describes Iris as the most genuinely modest person he had ever met, a modesty unaffected by being showered with honorary degrees or being made a Dame by the Queen. John writes that her sweetness of character remained as the Alzheimer's progressed. Astonishingly, he found that the disease brought them even closer together. He worried, in the book, about what might happen to her if he died first (mercifully, she has since died before him). In the face of Alzheimer's, they created a new marriage. He writes: 'After more than 40 years of taking marriage for granted, marriage has decided it is tired of this. Our marriage is now getting somewhere.' The original marriage may have finished, but their love story endures.

I would love to be able to write that everyone with Alzheimer's could ride the storm like Iris Murdoch, and that their carers could manage as well as John Bayley, but they are obviously exceptional. For most of us, Alzheimer's is a disaster with which it is very difficult to come to terms, that poses a myriad of problems for patient and carer alike.

One thing we can learn from these cases is that it hits anyone. I've reported meetings on Alzheimer's disease at which learned professors pontificated that if you keep your brain active when you are young, you have a better chance of avoiding Alzheimer's when you are older. Yet the disease hits people of all educational levels – no-one could have had a higher intellectual life than Iris Murdoch. Maybe it's a bit easier to hide your dwindling mental powers for a while if you start off brilliant than if you have had a limited education, so that it takes longer for the symptoms to be recognized.

I remember one meeting in which a researcher proposed that if you keep your brain active you can put off or slow down its decline. So I asked its chairman, Professor Zaven S. Khachaturian, at that time head of research into ageing at the US Institutes of Health in Bethesda, Maryland, how I could go about keeping my brain active. Would doing a different crossword every day be useful? He said it might, but only if it were in a second or third language. Doing it in my native English would not be enough! Even then, a foreign languge crossword might just give my brain the impetus it needed, but it still wouldn't guarantee protection against Alzheimer's. I'll have to learn the new language first, before I can try foreign crosswords. I don't think I've got enough years ahead of me to do so.

I'm still not sure whether or not Zaven, who is fluent in many European languges, was serious or had his tongue firmly in cheek. But he did make a further point: the evidence remains that we must all work very hard at keeping ourselves mentally agile, giving our brains a daily challenge. That should not stop if we develop dementia. Crucial to its management is the need to keep its sufferers mentally as well as physically active, and to help them play their part in normal everyday life for as long as possible. It may not slow the progress of the dementia, but it does make the quality of life better for both sufferer and carer.

12

Non-Alzheimer's dementias

Alzheimer's, the commonest form of dementia, has been described fully in previous chapters. Alzheimer's accounts for around two-thirds of the cases of dementia in North America and Europe. The last few chapters describing modern management of dementia relate mainly to Alzheimer's disease, but they are still relevant to the other forms of dementia. Once dementia has been definitely diagnosed, all the services for improving the person's life can be switched on, regardless of the underlying type. This includes the involvement of the Alzheimer's Society (see Chapter 6), which, despite its name, is dedicated to helping anyone with any form of dementia.

Non-Alzheimer's dementias include:
1 Vascular dementias
2 Diffuse Lewy body disease
3 Fronto-temporal dementia (including Pick's disease)
4 Other dementias:
    Alcohol-induced
    After head injury
    Linked to Parkinson's disease
    Linked to AIDS
    Creuzfeldt-Jakob disease
    Huntington's disease
    Others

Vascular dementia is responsible for about one in five cases of dementia among people of European origin. The accepted way to differentiate it from Alzheimer's is to use yet another scale – the Hachinski scale, developed by Professor Hachinski, of New York. It allocates numbers to sections such as abrupt onset; progression in steps, rather than gradually; physical complaints; swings in emotions; past high blood pressure or stroke; and signs of nervous system problems such as bouts of temporary blindness, weakness or numbness. A score of 0 to 4 suggests Alzheimer's and 5 to 12, vascular dementia or dementia of both types together.

The Hachinski score is calculated as shown in Table 12.1.

Table 12.1 The Hachinski score

Symptom	Score
Sudden onset	2
Stepwise deterioration	2
Physical complaints	1
Emotional swings	1
Past high blood pressure	1
Past stroke	1
Neurological symptoms	2
Neurological signs	2

Note: Alzheimer's = 0 to 4 Vascular = 5 to 12

The Hachinski score is not perfect, and in many cases the dementia has elements of both diseases, so differentiating between the two is often academic, especially as their treatment is largely similar. However, people with vascular dementia need treatment for their circulation problems as well as their dementia: this may mean something as simple as an aspirin a day or a drug to lower blood pressure, but it matters.

Diffuse Lewy body disease is the second commonest type of dementia. It is called this from microscopic changes in the brain that are specific to it. It is defined as dementia for at least six months, along with periods of confusion and hallucinations (patients with this form of dementia tend more than others to see things). They fall a lot, and show odd neurological signs such as rigid muscles, and they move more slowly and much less than normal. People with Lewy body dementia are over-sensitive to drugs for mental illness, and they deteriorate much faster than the average person with Alzheimer's disease.

The third major type of dementia is fronto-temporal disease. This refers to the areas of brain mainly affected. People with this type of dementia keep their memory until late in the illness. Their main early change is in their personality. They combine apathy with irritability, a strange misplaced jocularity and cheerfulness, with loss of normal tact and manners, linked with loss of concern about the feelings of others. They show lack of normal judgement and have no insight into their problems. They find language difficult, being unable to recall important words, and talking around a subject, rather than addressing it directly. One well-known feature of fronto-temporal dementia is the repetition of anecdotes or jokes interminably – it has even been given the name 'gramophone syndrome'. There may well be an increased sex drive, which in view of the personality changes is seen by others as very inappropriate.

Fronto-temporal dementia starts younger than Alzheimer's, and about one case in five is inherited. It includes Pick's disease, so called because the brain cells show large ballooned nerve cells named after their discoverer, Professor Pick. However, many people with fronto-temporal dementia do not show Pick's changes.

Other relatively common dementias are induced by excess alcohol, develop after a head injury, are linked to Huntington's disease, Parkinson's disease, to acquired immune deficiency syndrome (AIDS) and Creuzfeldt-Jakob disease (CJD). More than one hundred other types of dementia have been described in the medical literature, most of them single reports of particular syndromes linked to brain degeneration, but their management remains the same as that of Alzheimer's disease.

13

A non-medical approach

All that you have read so far is based on the medical model of dementia – the one that doctors use for assessing the illness and for making decisions about its long-term management. But there is another model of dementia which may be more practical, because it aims at assessing each individual person's needs and how to go about satisfying them. The main proponents of this model in my country, Scotland, are at Stirling University, where the dementia team is led by Professor Mary Marshall, director of the Dementia Services Development Centre. There are other centres throughout Britain. You will find your nearest through the Alzheimer's Society.

The aim is to extend and improve services, and to be a bridge between research and the front line. Professor Marshall initially trained in social work, and worked with people with dementia and their carers in Britain before going to Australia in 1982. There she discovered the positive approach, and a social model of care for people with dementia, that did not then exist in Britain. The Australians had embraced a non-medical model of services in the 1970s for all psychiatric fields, and dementia was included in it. This model became for Professor Marshall an important other half of the dementia story, separate from the usual doctor/nursing management.

Professor Marshall and the people she calls her 'incredible team' have come to believe that what is experienced by people with dementia is an impaired relationship between their brain and everything around them. She stresses that society, and most services, are not 'dementia friendly'. Much help for people with dementia, although well meaning, makes them more disabled. She wants to change that, and make sure that it is less devastating for them. Many of the problems that people with dementia experience can be minimized.

In effect, the brain is only half the story – dementia is all about people trying to communicate and trying to cope. She advises carers first on the 'built-in' environment. By that, she means the everyday environment around the home. As an example, people with dementia taken out of their usual environment become easily agitated. This is often because they do not know where the toilet is, and they fear that they will be caught short before they can find it. This fear can overpower all other thoughts, so that they are no longer listening to, or taking part in, all the social events and interactions with people around them. They seem distant to the rest of us, and this can be taken as just an inevitable, and untreatable, part of their dementia.

But the simple act of placing a sign in their full view to show where the toilet is can alter all that, by removing the anxiety, and allowing them to relax and start to communicate again. The same ploy can be used in the home. Loss of memory and disorientation can happen to people in their own home. This is what triggers the 'this is not my home' confusion described in Chapter 9. Making the doors in the house more like those they knew as young adults, for example, can ease confusion. Improving lighting is another ploy – the older eye sees much better in bright light. Using a familiar landmark as a focal point in the room is yet another strategy, as is putting signs up in the bedroom, toilet, kitchen and living area that clearly show where all one's familiar things are. Taken together, all these fairly simple changes can minimize the person's agitation, aggression and confusion. Not all may be needed: the solution varies from person to person.

This is what Professor Marshall calls 'making the environments in which patients find themselves orientating, and making familiar and necessary things speak to them'. She prefers to use the 'disability model of dementia' that focuses on the disabilities and not the cause, to find many ways to compensate for them.

Her centre does not work with relatives but with caring staff and volunteers, believing that the role of working with relatives should be left to carers organizations such as the Alzheimer's Society (in Scotland this is Alzheimer Scotland – Action on Dementia). All the useful societies and their addresses are listed in Chapter 16 at the end of this book. However, the material her centre produces helps professional caring staff and volunteers and relatives alike.

Professor Marshall does not see impaired memory as particularly dreadful. It only becomes bad when no-one around you understands what you are trying to say or recall, or can cope with your efforts to do so. 'If society were truly dementia friendly,' she says, 'it would not be such a big deal.'

The centre tries to teach people to listen to the emotion behind the confused words. One consequence of dementia is that sufferers find ordinary things difficult to put into words. Often when they say 'I must get the children from school' or 'My mother is expecting me' or when they are behaving oddly, what they are really meaning is 'I feel lost and bewildered. I need to be cared for and the security of knowing who I am.' Often what they want to say to their carers is too painful for them to admit or articulate. That is when carers can ask 'Are you feeling lost?' or, incongruously for an elderly person, but extremely relevantly, 'Do you miss your mum?'

Let's take the case of an elderly lady who seemed superficially to be back in time nearly 50 years, to the time when she was a young mother. She was continually looking for her baby, and complaining that she missed her. The staff in her nursing home tried giving her dolls and talking to her about babies and the birth of her own children. But what she was really missing was the physical contact and warmth that she had enjoyed with her babies. Once the staff sat and cuddled her, her need for her babies disappeared.

The Stirling Centre employs a poet, John Killick. He is a Research Fellow, working on communication through art, and is also writer in residence for Westminster Health Care. Using a poet to help people with dementia is not such a strange idea. John says that people with dementia talk in pictures and are poets themselves. Some of their behaviour comes from the difficulty they have in expressing the concept that they have a pain, or some other problem, so that they become restless or agitated or sick in an odd way. Carers who are with them much of the time often know when things aren't right with them. But it can be hard for a daughter, say, to stand back and accept that her mother is trying to tell her something, and to understand what is behind the rage and frustration.

This can be done by using a form of communication other than normal conversation. John works with artists to encourage people with dementia to use paintings, sculptures, photographs, embroidery and poems to enhance their sense of well-being, and to improve their communication with their families and carers. The arts, he says, are a great vehicle for self-expression, whether it is banging a drum, painting a picture or creating a poem.

Anyone who has cared for someone with dementia will recognize these case histories. Professor Marshall believes that they stem from the fact that what they are trying to say is so personal and difficult for them that they have to employ simpler ideas to express their current needs. They may have to be drawn from memories of long past times, such as when they needed to care for someone else.

Professor Marshall's centre is producing a CD-ROM and will produce a book for general practitioners on understanding behaviour in dementia. Until now, the quick solution has been 'here's the tablets': Professor Marshall stresses that the aim is to provide doctors and carers with a 'bag full of other tricks to offer, as well'.

The Stirling Centre has a consultancy staff team, research staff, and a training officer with a team of associate trainers, four general practitioners, two community nurses, an occupational therapist and two social workers. Psychiatrists and other staff join the team regularly. They also have people with dementia as advisers. Just because you have dementia certainly does not stop you from making valuable contributions to its understanding and management. Two of the researchers spend much of their working lives talking to people with dementia.

This team promotes an extremely helpful system for assessing the personal needs of people with dementia. Called CarenapD (Care Needs Assessment Pack for Dementia) it is essentially non-medical. It is not based on an interview with people with dementia, but on discussions with them, their carers and other professionals. It has seven areas of study:

- Health and mobility
- Social interaction
- Self-care and toilet
- Behaviour and mental state
- Thinking and memory
- Housecare
- Living in the community.

Each of these areas has a page with subdivisions that are individually assessed, and their needs analysed. For example, under 'Health and mobility' the subdivisions are:

- physical health
- diarrhoea and/or constipation
- state of feet (not mobility)
- hearing
- walking on level ground
- steps and stairs

- balance and falls
- getting in and out of a chair
- getting in and out of bed.

Each subdivision is then ticked as 'no need', 'met need' or 'unmet need', and the action to be taken to meet any unmet need is noted accordingly. This ranges from minor help, such as providing eye care or chiropody, to more specialist assessment.

Its primary aim is to prompt creative thinking about the most appropriate type of help for each aspect of the illness. It should help to organize the optimum care for each individual. CarenapD, however, has had an added use that will help whole communities. By summing the results for many dementia sufferers in one area it has alerted the teams looking after them to the commonest problems and to ways of solving them. Applying CarenapD has allowed local authorities and nursing and medical teams to plan ahead much more efficiently to meet the needs of all their clients with dementia.

By August 1999 CarenapD had been licensed to 17 users, predominantly in Scotland, with some in Northern Ireland and England. Most of the licensees were in Social Work Departments, Health Boards and Trusts, Voluntary Organizations, and Primary Health Care Teams. However, its use is expanding rapidly. Anyone wishing to know more about it should contact Alan Chapman, Training Officer at e-mail *a.j.chapman@stir.ac.uk* Information on the CarenapD software programme is available from James B. Grant at *j.b.grant@stir.ac.uk*

Professor Marshall's message is one of hope. There is much, she says, that can be done to help people with dementia and their families. Much has already been done. After many years in this post, Professor Marshall finds the improvement in dementia services amazing because, up until relatively recently, people with dementia were assumed to have porridge in their heads. There is now a revolution in the approach to dementia that has received hardly any acknowledgement in the medical press. The focus is now on the remaining competence of people with dementia, and not on their failing abilities. Everyone has potential that needs to be realized.

I am inclined to agree with her. As an orthodox family doctor, I have often despaired in my management of elderly people with dementia, because I did not have the time or the means or knowledge to develop the expertise to treat them properly. Nor did I have any support from the medical authorities. It seemed that the only management was to keep people at home as long as possible, and to admit them to hospital care when their physical state or their behaviour made further home care impossible. During their stay at home, little could be offered except a form of 'babysitting' and drugs to minimize the behaviour problems. That usually meant sedation.

That is all changing. As attitudes like Professor Marshall's spread, doctors and carers will find that there is plenty to be done, and more expertise to be drawn upon. The upwards curve in understanding and caring for people with dementia is an ever-steeper one, and it will continue to rise.

Unfortunately, many relatives of people with dementia still experience poor services, indifferent general practitioners (many have too little time to concentrate on what they see as the elderly with chronic mental illness), and third-rate nursing homes. However, the problems posed by dementia are now much better understood and ways of coping with them are being worked out. Now the onus is on people everywhere to be given the chance to put them into practice.

Professor Marshall emphasizes the need for carers, families and people with dementia themselves to be assertive. 'Don't let anyone brush you off with statements like nothing can be done,' she says. Her fundamental message is optimistic. The centre supports training that uses people with dementia to provide 'input'. Jean, a woman with dementia, is helping a local dementia initiative by contributing to the training of their staff. Jean's audience always listens avidly.

I asked Professor Marshall if putting her caring approach into action not only eased the patients' torment of minds but also might slow down progress of dementia. She accepted that this is the thousand dollar question. The late Professor Tom Kitwood, of Bradford, who wrote the book *Dementia Reconsidered*, discussed the possibility of rementia – in theory, the reversal of dementia, if the lines of communication, so obviously cut in dementia, could be reconnected. Whether this could ever be achieved simply by improving people's social environment so that they can enjoy full communication and understanding with their carers and family again remains to be seen.

Even if rementia is just a dream, Tom Kitwood's attitudes to dementia were still enlightening in a speciality that is highly geared towards medicines and nursing care. In his obituary in January 1999, his close colleague, Errolyn Bruce, wrote:

He believed that it was impossible for any one person to meet fully the emotional needs of someone with dementia. He once estimated that to give people with dementia all the care and stimulation they need, without leaving their carers drained and depleted, it would need a team of seven dedicated and committed people supporting each person with dementia. Tom believed that caring for a person with dementia requires enormous reserves of sensitivity, patience and creativity – qualities that are particularly hard to sustain in the face of the progressive loss of a significant relationship.

Tom Kitwood, having had a lonely childhood himself (he was sent to boarding school when he was seven), identified strongly with the feelings of loss and abandonment of people with dementia, and noticed that their reasonable feelings about their predicament were seldom recognized by their carers. Their family sees their anger and frustration as part of the dementia, rather than a normal response to loss. Tom, like Mary Marshall, stressed the need to look at the person rather than the disease. He looked on people with dementia as people with a disability, and not as victims of a disease who had become non-persons or shadows of their former selves. Only by doing that can they be given the best possible quality of life for their circumstances.

Professor Marshall strongly agrees with this approach to dementia. It may prevent a lot of pain and anguish, she says, even though in the end it does not 'prevent the grey cells from packing in'. (However, many European specialists in dementia are into memory training, and they believe that this can at least maintain brain function for some months, and perhaps lead to slower deterioration.)

The downside to this approach to dementia care is that it is all very hard work, especially for carers. They must look after themselves, physically and mentally. They must recharge their batteries regularly, and learn survival skills. Many carers burn out from the constant stress and strain. Eventually there comes a stage when enough is enough. Professor Marshall supports the British tradition that in the final stages tender loving care is all that can and should be applied. There should be no radical interventions.

Even in those stages, people with dementia need relief from other causes of pain and distress. One elderly lady in a nursing home, but not yet in the terminal stages of her disease, had repeated bowel blockages, needing surgery. The surgeon refused to operate, because of her dementia, and she died. This is an illustration of the 'knee jerk' reaction of some parts of the health care system, that 'dementia equals poor quality of life, equals let people die'. Her nurses knew that she still had much enjoyment in life, that her blockage was causing her distress, and that with surgery she could have 'bounced back' into her previously happy personality for a few more months. This case is not uncommon. There is always the danger, Professor Marshall says, that the acute sector staff who do not know such people well will assume that it is not worth treating them purely because they have dementia.

All decisions about the management of dementia must take the quality of the person's life into account. Even in the final stages this can be reasonable, especially when there is excellent professional care. There is often too much emphasis on scores, failures in performance and other negative aspects of the disease, and not enough on the positive things that can be done. This, above all, is what people like Professor Marshall and her team wish to change.

14

Caring for the carers

If you are a carer, this chapter is for you. Faced with years of looking after someone with dementia, it is natural for you to feel huge stresses – grief, guilt, anger, even aggression are all normal reactions to being placed in this awful position. There is solid evidence that carers are much more likely than the rest of the population to have psychological problems and depression. Australian, American and British researchers have all reported high levels of depression in people caring for persons with dementia. Carers' physical health is also threatened: if they have had high blood pressure before becoming carers it increases afterwards.

Caring for someone with dementia can cause people to become isolated from friends, because they do not know how to relate to the new conditions within the family, and are frightened by the disease. No-one likes to visit regularly a house in which carer and patient are living in obviously strained conditions, so many friendships melt away. At the same time, many carers have to give up most of their social activities. Memberships of health or sports clubs and other hobbies are given up, making the isolation even more acute. Often the job has to go, and another group of friends is lost. Caring eventually takes up every waking moment.

There are also financial costs that can become crippling. In Britain medical and nursing care is free, up to a point. But when extra care is needed, it often has to be found privately, and that can be very expensive. Residential nursing care can take all but a few thousand pounds of the family savings, and it is often impossible for the carer to go back to work to retrieve them. In all these stressful circumstances, many carers neglect their own health, to the extent that they sometimes ignore early warning signs of serious disease in themselves until it is too late. And if that makes the carer worried and anxious, these emotions are transferred to the patient, whose behaviour worsens accordingly.

Younger carers are more at risk from the stress of caring than older ones, and men carers are more at risk than women. This is particularly true if the carer has had a depressive illness in the past, and reacts oddly to the initial news of the dementia (such as denying the possibility). Carers fare worse, too, when their previous relationship with the patient was poor, or when they have a conflict of interest within the family. The archetypal example of the last is when a married daughter has to spend more time caring for a parent than for her husband and children.

Carers who do better are usually mature in their abilities to solve problems, know how to manage problems 'on the hoof', and have taken the trouble to learn about dementia. So if you have read this book through to this page, you have almost certainly made yourself a better carer and will avoid some emotional problems. Other plus points that help carers cope are a good previous relationship between you and your patient, plenty of social support from family and friends, membership of a self-help group for Alzheimer's and continuing to keep up hobbies and a good social life.

Some carers go so far in their frustration with their lot that they physically abuse their dementing relations. Such 'elder abusers' are usually isolated, under great stress, have little support and may themselves be alcohol abusers. They need help, not punishment, but the people they have abused must be removed from their care, for both their sakes.

It is almost normal, however, for carers to feel angry and resentful and to contemplate violence. One study reported that one in five of 236 carers for dementing relatives felt violent towards them, and another third of them had gone so far as to become violent. Such feelings can be assuaged at least in part by education, not just of the carers themselves, but of the whole family, about dementia and the problems it poses. They must learn about:

- legal and financial problems;
- considerations of psychological reactions to the diagnosis and to the later deterioration;
- counselling of the family about conflicts and the need not to neglect other family members;
- joining support groups and learning how to use their expertise;
- the need for respite care of all types;
- learning management skills from books, videos and support group meetings;
- keeping fit and getting fast medical care for any illness in the carer;
- how to deal with a patient who refuses to co-operate.

There is, as yet, no cure or satisfactory treatment for dementia, but carers can achieve a lot of satisfaction from a job well done, and a loved person who was cared for with love and expertise until the end. That thought can compensate at least a little for the years spent devoted, often selflessly, to such care.

15

People who can help

This is an appropriate place to describe the ways in which the community services, official and voluntary, can help. Need for these services grows through the middle stages of dementia, and comes to a peak just before the final stages, when 24-hour care, preferably in a nursing home setting is usually needed.

Systems of care in the community for people with dementia differ from country to country, and even within countries. Some countries spend a lot of public money on dementia care, others spend very little. Most earmark a mixture of private and public funds for it, and in many of them the proportion spent from public funds on each individual depends on the patient's ability to pay.

However the schemes are funded, most have many features in common. Nurses visit homes to help with drugs, personal care, mobility, and whatever skilled nursing is needed. They are also an excellent source of advice to carers and will take progress reports back to the family doctors. Some systems allow non-nursing personal care assistants to bathe and wash patients.

Occupational therapists help to organize the home, making it easier for the carers and patients to perform everyday tasks that have become beyond them. They can provide practical aids for washing and the toilet, help carers to plan their home care efficiently, and provide relevant and achievable activities for the person with dementia to occupy their time.

Physiotherapists will visit to assess and treat the patient's physical difficulties, such as difficulties with muscles and joints and lack of mobility. As the dementia progresses, limbs can become fixed in semi-bent positions, and one task of physiotherapists is to prevent such 'contractures' by stretching them regularly. Speech therapists may be asked to review problems with formulating words and swallowing, but they often encounter difficulties because of the patient's inability to co-operate fully.

Probably more relevant are the social services, such as the British 'Meals on Wheels'. This ensures that the patient has a wholesome cooked meal every day. Nowadays, it can usually be organized to cater for ethnic, dietary and religious preferences. Home helps clean, do the housework and may even cook. Local councils will help to maintain gardens and do home repairs, and provide transport to day centres, doctors' offices and hospital appointments.

All these services remove a huge burden from carers, and they should take advantage of them. The carer who manages to get regular respite, from a home-sitter for a regular evening, or one day a week in the day centre, or for a week or fortnight in a nursing home once or twice a year, is much better able to shoulder the burden than the one who struggles on, 52 weeks of the year. Remember that creaking gate.

Carers desperately need respite, yet it seems to be the service that local authorities most often fail to provide adequately. Sometimes that is due to patients reacting badly against alternative carers, and the carers not wishing to upset them. Sometimes it is purely financial – the family cannot afford it. But most of the time, it is because there are too few places in day centres or nursing homes for them. Only pressure from the public and the Alzheimer's Associations can improve that.

Patients reluctant to go to day centres may be persuaded to go by the doctor suggesting that contact with the staff there can help their memory and brain power. There is no proof that it does, but it removes from the carer the 'you do not want to care for me' accusation.

As for spending a week or more in respite care in a nursing home, it often takes several visits before the patient accepts that this is a regular and beneficial part of the treatment. It also prepares the way for permanent nursing home stay, so that it is best, if possible, to use for respite the nursing home into which you plan to place the patient when this becomes necessary. If it has become a 'home from home' by the time that decision is made, the patient is much more likely to accept it with no fuss.

16

Important addresses

Alzheimer's disease

A host of people and organizations are dedicated to helping families with Alzheimer's. In this chapter, I list as many as I can with their addresses and phone numbers. I may have missed a few in your own area, but your local Alzheimer's Society branch is bound to have comprehensive knowledge of who and where they are. These organizations will transform the life of any carers who are struggling along on their own.

The first name has to be the **Alzheimer's Society**, which supports carers with a wide range of services, including sitters and respite. You will meet local members and share information and ways of solving problems, receive advice sheets and a monthly newsletter, and you may qualify for a financial grant from their Caring Fund.

The Alzheimer's Society is concerned for people with any form of dementia and their carers, so that if the problem is vascular dementia or Creuzfeldt-Jakob disease, you will still be welcome. The Society has invested more than £2 million in research into the causes of and possible cures for dementia, a sum that is growing. Its headquarters in the United Kingdom are at:
Devon House
58 St Katharine's Way
London E1W 1JX
Telephone: 020 7423 3500
Website: www.alzheimers.org.uk
Email: enquiries@alzheimers.org.uk

In Scotland, the sister organization is **Alzheimer Scotland Action on Dementia**. Its details are:
22 Drumsheugh Gardens
Edinburgh EH3 7RN
24-hour helpline: 0808 808 3000
Website: www.alzscot.org
Email: alzheimer@alzscot.org

The Dementia Resource Centre has many local projects, listed in local telephone directories. Its headquarters are at:
32 Riccartsbar Avenue
Paisley PA2 6BG
Telephone: 0141 887 4902

Alzheimer Scotland also strongly supports the **Dementia Services Development Centre** (DSDC, see Chapter 13), which has set up similar centres throughout Britain, and will provide information about those in your area. The DSDC can be contacted at:
The University of Stirling
Stirling FK9 4LA
Telephone: 01786 467740
Website: www.dementia.stir.ac.uk
Email: dementia@stir.ac.uk

Non-Alzheimer's dementia

Several organizations cater for people with particular types of dementia. The **Huntington's Disease Association** helps families with this disease, and has a network of local support groups throughout the country. Its headquarters are at:
Down Stream Building
1 London Bridge
London SE1 9BG
Telephone: 020 7022 1950
Website: www.hda.org.uk
Email: info@hda.org.uk

The **Scottish Huntington's Association** is at:
Thistle House
61 Main Road
Elderslie
Paisley PA5 9BA
Telephone: 01505 322245
Website: www.hdscotland.org
Email: sha-admin@hdscotland.org

The Parkinson's Disease Society of the UK is very aware of the connections between Parkinson's disease and Alzheimer's and supports research that covers subjects common to both illnesses. The Society's headquarters are at:
215 Vauxhall Bridge Road
London SW1V 1EJ
Telephone: 020 7931 8080
Helpline Mon.–Fri., 9.30 a.m.–5.30 p.m.: 0808 800 0303
Website: www.parkinsons.org.uk
Email: enquiries@parkinsons.org.uk

Families of people with AIDS-related dementia can contact the **Terrence Higgins Trust** at:
314–320 Gray's Inn Road
London WC1X 8DP
Telephone: 020 7812 1600
Helpline: 0845 122 1200
Website: www.tht.org.uk
Email: info@tht.org.uk

Advice and support for carers

Every district in the United Kingdom has an **Age Concern** organization. Age Concern provides services such as day centres, relatives' groups and shopping schemes. The staff advise on other local services and benefits. I particularly like their profusion of books and pamphlets, well written and easily read, on every aspect of care for dementia patients and their families. Age Concern's main bases are:

Age Concern England
Astral House
1268 London Road
London SW16 4ER
Telephone: 020 8765 7200
Freephone 8 a.m.–7 p.m.: 0800 00 99 66
Website: www.ageconcern.org.uk
Email: ace@ace.org.uk

Age Concern Cymru (Wales)
Ty John Pathy
13–14 Neptune Court
Vanguard Way
Cardiff CF24 5PJ
Telephone: 029 2043 1555
Freephone 8 a.m.–7 p.m.: 0800 00 99 66
Website: www.accymru.org.uk
Email: enquiries@accymru.org.uk

Age Concern Northern Ireland
3 Lower Crescent
Belfast BT7 1NR
Telephone: 028 9024 5729
Freephone 8 a.m.–7 p.m.: 0800 00 99 66
Website: www.ageconcernni.org
Email: info@ageconcernni.org

Age Concern Scotland
Causewayside House
160 Causewayside
Edinburgh EH9 1PR
Telephone: 0131 220 3345
Freephone 7 a.m.–7 p.m.: 0800 00 99 66
Website: www.ageconcernscotland.org.uk
Email: enquiries@acscot.org.uk

Another favourite organization for dementia sufferers is the **Crossroads Care Attendant Scheme**. Your phone book will have the number of your nearest Crossroads group. I thoroughly recommend the Crossroads teams: all their Care Attendants seem to have been handpicked for their cheerfulness, inexhaustible physical strength and vast patience. They are wonderful. Crossroads English headquarters is at:

Dunsmore Business Centre
Rugby
Warwickshire CV21 3HH
Telephone: 01788 532512
Email: rugby.crossroads@care4free.net

Carers UK tries to help people whose lives are restricted by their need to look after someone else, whatever the affliction. It provides advice and a newsletter. The English branch is at:
32–36 Loman Street
London SE1 0EE
Telephone: 020 7922 8000
CarersLine: 0808 808 7777 Weds/Thurs 10 a.m.–12 p.m./2 p.m–4 p.m.
Website: www.carersuk.org
Email: info@carersuk.org

The Scottish address is:
91 Mitchell Street
Glasgow G1 3LN
Telephone: 0141 221 9141
Website: www.carerscotland.org
Email: info@carerscotland.org

Cruse Bereavement Care gives free and confidential advice on bereavement to older people and carers. The English address is:
PO Box 800
Richmond
Surrey TW9 1RG
Telephone: 020 8939 9530 (administration)
Helpline: 0844 477 9400
Website: www.crusebereavementcare.org.uk
Email: helpline@crusebereavementcare.org.uk

The Scottish address is:
Riverview House
Friarton Road
Perth PH2 8DF
Telephone: 01738 444 178
Website: www.crusescotland.org
Email: info@www.crusescotland.org

The Disabled Living Foundation helps carers by providing special aids, such as wheelchairs, incontinence pads and commodes, and advice on how to cope with physical disabilities. Its English headquarters are at:

380–384 Harrow Road
London W9 2HU
Telephone: 020 7289 6111
Helpline: 0845 130 9177
Website: www.dlf.org.uk

In Scotland, contact:
Advice Service Capability Scotland (ASCS)
11 Ellersly Road
Edinburgh EH12 6HY
Telephone: 0131 313 5510
Website: www.capability-scotland.org.uk
Email: ascs@capability-scotland.org.uk

Disability Alliance publishes the *Disability Rights Handbook*, a guide to financial benefits and services for anyone with a disability. Disability Alliance is at:
1st Floor East
Universal House
88–94 Wentworth Street
London E1 7SA
Telephone: 020 7247 8776
Website: www.disabilityalliance.org

Your local **Citizens' Advice Bureau** can provide advice on particular problems. The address and telephone number will be in your local directory. The national CAB headquarters are at:
115–123 Pentonville Road
London N1 9LZ

MIND, formerly the National Association for Mental Health, publishes booklets on problems in dementia, and has active local groups in many areas, the addresses and phone numbers are in local directories. Its headquarters are at:
Granta House
15–19 Broadway
Stratford
London E15 4BQ
Telephone: 020 8519 2122
MindinfoLine: 0845 766 0163 (Monday to Friday, 9.15 a.m.–5.15 p.m.)

Website: www.mind.org.uk
Email: contact@mind.org.uk

Local community health councils are happy to hear from carers. They are a fund of useful information on local hospital and community care services, and will listen to comments and complaints about them. Their addresses and phone numbers are in local directories.

Holiday and respite care

Some organizations help to provide holidays for carers and their people with special needs, such as dementia. One is **Holiday Care** at:
Tourism for All
The Hawkins Suite
Enham Place
Enham Alamein
Andover SP11 6JS
Telephone: 0845 124 9971
Website: www.holidaycare.org.uk
Email: info@holidaycare.org

Vitalise (formerly the **Winged Fellowship Trust**) provides holidays and respite care for severely disabled people, with and without escorts. Vitalise can be contacted at:
12 City Forum
250 City Road
London EC1V 8AF
Telephone: 0845 345 1972
Website: www.vitalise.org.uk
Email: info@vitalise.org.uk

Advice about nursing homes and residential care

Other organizations can provide details of nursing homes and residential care for people with dementia. One is **Elderly Accommodation Counsel** (**EAC**), which has a database on such services throughout the United Kingdom. It does not inspect the nursing

homes, so potential customers are well advised to see them themselves before making decisions. EAC can be contacted at:
Third Floor
89 Albert Embankment
London SE1 7TP
Advice line: 020 7820 1343
Website: www.housingcare.org
　　　　www.eac.org.uk

Grace Consulting gives details of private homes that they assess. They are at:
Orchard House
Albury
Guildford
Surrey GU5 9AG
Telephone: 0800 137 669
Website: www.graceconsulting.co.uk
Email: enquiries@graceconsulting.co.uk

The Registered Nursing Home Association provides information on all registered UK nursing homes. The Association can be found at:
John Hewitt House
Tunnel Lane
Off Lifford Lane
Kings Norton
Birmingham B30 3JN
Telephone: 0121 451 1088
Website: www.rnha.co.uk
Email: info@rnha.co.uk

Help in the community

Finally, many voluntary organizations are interested in offering help to people in their communities with dementia. This has always been a main interest of local religious groups, Christian, Muslim, and Hindu. Dementia crosses all barriers, and unites people of all religions in the fight against it.

Then there are men's and women's local groups, such as the

Rotary, the Round Table, Inner Wheel, Lions' Clubs, Women's Guilds, Women's Institutes, Mothers' Union, Soroptimists, Samaritans, Hospital Leagues of Friends, Pensioners' Action Groups, and so on. They are all interested in helping carers and people with chronic illnesses in their districts. If you have a contact with one of these groups, don't be afraid or ashamed to use it.

I started this book as a family doctor with only the same relatively limited experience of caring for people with Alzheimer's as any other busy general practitioner. It was only while doing the extra research for it that I came to realize how much had improved in Alzheimer's care in the past few years. And how many more people are able, and willing, to help. And how much research is going on to improve not only the treatment of the disease, but also the many people with it, and their carers.

With all this goodwill and attention, things can only get better. I am confident we will see great strides in our understanding of all the dementias in the twenty-first century, and in ways to reverse and perhaps even cure them. We are only just starting to manage dementias properly. Think of where medicine stood only 50 years ago, and imagine how it might evolve in the next 50 years.

References

Brotchie, Jane, *Caring for Someone Who Has Dementia*, London, Age Concern Books, 2003.

Cayton, Harry *et al.*, *Dementia: Alzheimer's and Other Dementias at Your Fingertips*, London, Class Publishing, 2002.

Feil, Naomi, *The Validation Breakthrough: Simple Techniques for Communicating with People with Alzheimer's-Type Dementia*, Baltimore, Health Professions Press, 2002.

Grant, Linda, *Remind Me Who I Am, Again*, London, Granta Books, 1999.

Koenig-Coste, Joanne, *Learning to Speak Alzheimer's: The New Approach to Living Positively with Alzheimer's Disease*, London, Vermilion, 2003.

Marriott, Hugh, *The Selfish Pig's Guide to Caring*, Clifton-upon-Teme, Worcestershire, Polperro Heritage Press, 2003.

Woolf, Josephine and Michael, *Is the Cooker Turned Off? Caring for an Older Person with Failing Memory*, Oxton, Wirral, Gorselands Publishing, 2003.

Index